Social Work Practice in Community-Based Health Care

THE HAWORTH PRESS®
Titles of Related Interest

Social Work Practice in Community-Based Health Care

Marcia Egan, PhD
Goldie Kadushin, PhD

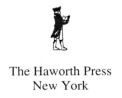

The Haworth Press
New York

For more information on this book or to order, visit
http://www.haworthpress.com/store/product.asp?sku=5273

or call 1-800-HAWORTH (800-429-6784) in the United States and Canada
or (607) 722-5857 outside the United States and Canada
or contact orders@HaworthPress.com

The Haworth Press, Inc. 10 Alice Street, Binghamton, NY 13904-1580.

PUBLISHER'S NOTE
The development, preparation, and publication of this work has been undertaken with great care. However, the Publisher, employees, editors, and agents of The Haworth Press are not responsible for any errors contained herein or for consequences that may ensue from use of materials or information contained in this work. The Haworth Press is committed to the dissemination of ideas and information according to the highest standards of intellectual freedom and the free exchange of ideas. Statements made and opinions expressed in this publication do not necessarily reflect the views of the Publisher, Directors, management, or staff of The Haworth Press, Inc., or an endorsement by them.

Cover design by Kerry E. Mack.

Library of Congress Cataloging-in-Publication Data

Egan, Marcia.
    Social work practice in community-based health care / Marcia Egan, Goldie Kadushin.
        p. cm.
    ISBN: 978-0-7890-2566-1 (hard : alk. paper)
    ISBN: 978-0-7890-2567-8 (soft : alk. paper)
    1. Medical social work—United States. 2. Ambulatory medical care—United States. 3. Community-based social services—United States. 4. Community health services—United States. I. Kadushin, Goldie. II. Title.

HV687.5.U5E43 2007
362.1'0425—dc22

                                                                        2006033838

ABOUT THE AUTHORS

Marcia Egan, PhD, is Associate Professor in the College of Social Work at the University of Tennessee in Knoxville. She collaborates with the UT Institute on Women's Health in an interdisciplinary, community-based, maternal-child health project. Her research on social work health care practice and on resilience among marginalized women is published regularly in several leading peer-reviewed journals.

Goldie Kadushin, PhD, is Associate Professor in the Helen Bader School of Social Welfare at the University of Wisconsin-Milwaukee. She is coordinator of the UW-M Interdisciplinary Certificate in Applied Gerontology and is co-author of *Social Work Interview: A Guide for Human Service Professionals*.

CONTENTS

APPENDIXES

Preface

The profession of social work has a long history in the field of health care. Early on, health care social work took place largely in community settings with attention on the interactions of economic and social factors and health. During the intervening decades, health care social work moved largely out of the community into hospitals centering on individual factors. Recently, however, as a result of the paradigm shift in health, social workers are called to reenter the community and to do so with new health care practice knowledge and skills in emerging and innovative settings. The purpose of this text is to provide the knowledge and skills pertinent to social work in the current environment of community-based health care. Community-based health care, also referred to as ambulatory health care, social work in this book is differentiated from both inpatient/institutional/hospital care and from care delivered in the home, such as hospice and home health.

The requisite knowledge and skills reflect several ongoing factors, including rapid advances in the technologies of medical care and communication, the dominance of managed care, and the increasing diversity of the health care consumer population. Skills in time-limited, evidence-based direct practice and in practice on behalf of consumer populations are essential. In aggregate, knowledge and skills are informed by the disparities in health status and access to care, and by the empirically evidenced links between economic and psychosocial characteristics and behavior in the etiology of several major prevalent diseases.

The content of this book results from an analysis of the literature with specific criteria for inclusion. These criteria were that the knowledge, concepts, and skills are from literature that is as current as possible, empirically based, and pertinent specifically for best practice in ambulatory health care social work. In a few instances, content includes literature not meeting those criteria because these provide an

Social Work Practice in Community-Based Health Care
© 2007 by The Haworth Press, Inc. All rights reserved.
doi:10.1300/5273_a

excellent conceptual or seminal discussion of a topic and/or accurate history.

The book is organized into three parts. Part I supplies the context of ambulatory health care social work in chapters on the revolution in funding and delivery (Chapter 1), the evolving trends and health care needs of the consumer population (Chapter 2), and a conceptual framework for culturally competent practice (Chapter 3). Part I concludes with a discussion of the nature of social work in ambulatory health, a brief history of health care social work, prevalent and emerging settings for practice with related approaches, public health perspectives, and the use of new communication technologies in practice (Chapter 4). Part II provides knowledge, concepts, and skills for evidence-based practice directly with consumers (Chapter 5) and practice on behalf of consumer groups and populations (Chapter 6), with consumer scenarios included throughout. Part II concludes with an overview of appropriate methods and their applications in evaluating direct practice and programs on behalf of populations of consumers (Chapter 7). Each chapter begins with an inbox presentation of the questions that the chapter addresses and concludes with discussion questions/activities and a glossary of terms. Ethical considerations are examined throughout the chapters.

In the third part, Appendix A provides four exemplars of current community-based health care programs for culturally diverse and/or at-risk populations that demonstrate the concepts and skills explored in the previous chapters. Appendix B is a summary of Web sites that were found by critical analysis to provide up-to-date and useful information and resources for culturally responsive practice in ambulatory health social work. Appendix C is a consolidation of the conceptual framework presented in Chapter 3 for culturally competent practice (Chapter 3) in outline form of topics and issues for assessment.

The process of writing this text was challenging and intriguing— challenging because of the scope and volume of relevant knowledge and empirically based skills, and intriguing because of the consistently emergent new knowledge and skills to inform practice in ambulatory health care arenas that are in themselves evolving. It is our hope that readers are also intrigued, and the text gives both shape and substance to social work in ambulatory health care in the twenty-first century.

PART I:
THE CONTEXT
OF COMMUNITY-BASED
HEALTH CARE

Chapter 1

The Revolution in Health Care Funding and Delivery

- *What prompted the revolution in health care funding?*
- *What is the history of health care funding in the United States?*
- *What is "managed care"?*
- *What are the ethical considerations related to health care funding?*
- *How does managed care influence community-based social work health care practice?*

INTRODUCTION

The recent paradigm shift in health care transformed the locus (where), the structure (how), and the focus (to whom) of health care delivery (Dziegielewski & Holliman, 2001; Gorin, 2003). The revolution in health care funding contributing to the paradigm shift was largely driven by the continual rising health care costs over the last two decades of the twentieth century. Several factors interacted to contribute to those increasing costs, including

- the increasing number of older adults;
- the development and use of costly technological health care treatments;

Social Work Practice in Community-Based Health Care
© 2007 by The Haworth Press, Inc. All rights reserved.
doi:10.1300/5273_01

- an excess of empty hospital beds prompting hospitals to shift costs to existing patients;
- the unregulated nature of the health care and insurance industries.

Health care systems were fragmented and redundant, with gaps in needed services. That is, multiple providers delivered similar services to often-overlapping consumer populations while, also, not attending to unmet existing and/or emerging consumer needs for health care.

The annual cost of health care in the United States increased exponentially in the latter part of the twentieth century; projections are for continuing increases in the twenty-first century. By 1990, national health care expenditures approached $700 billion a year (Berkman, 1996). Between 1990 and 2000 the cost of health care in the United States nearly doubled, from $696 billion to $1,309 billion a year (Centers for Medicaid and Medicare Services, 2001, 2003). Estimates for annual health care costs are projected to be upward of $16 trillion by 2030 (Dziegielewski & Holliman, 2001). Strunk and Ginsburg (2004) and Gorin (2003) suggest that the main driver in the continuously increasing cost of health care is the advancement and usage of medical technology, a good deal of which is very expensive and which fosters new spending.

This chapter explores the history of rising costs and the attempts that were made to control those costs that led to the transformation of health care, the history of managing the delivery of health care in the United States, and the types and dynamics of managed health care systems. Each of these is discussed in the context of the impact of the paradigm shift in health care on social work practice in ambulatory health care, with special attention to the resulting ethical dilemmas.

CONTROLLING ESCALATING COSTS OF HEALTH CARE

Escalating costs and health insurer reports of large financial losses coupled with widespread hospital closures and empty beds prompted a series of reforms initiated in the early 1980s to control health care expenditures (Caputi & Heiss, 1984; Jensen, Morrisey, Gaffney, & Liston, 1997; Rosenberg, 1998; Shortell, Gillies, & Devers, 1995). Concerns to control hospital care costs specifically resulted in the development and implementation of the diagnosis related groups (DRGs) policies and regulations. The DRGs were based on the precept that reducing the duration of a patient's length of stay (LOS) in the hospital would reduce the cost of his or her hospitalization. Thus, the DRGs pursued cost containment for hospital care by limiting coverage to predetermined, fixed payments and to a predetermined duration of hospitalization for a given medical condition and diagnosis. The DRGs transformed hospital care funding procedures from the traditional physician-centered "fee for services rendered" reimbursement system to preset standardized payments (Caputi & Heiss, 1984). Switching accountability and coverage for hospital care from the physician to the hospital created a financial incentive for hospitals to limit the duration of inpatient care (Reamer, 1997).

However, the implementation of DRGs had two consequences beyond just reducing the LOS. The first consequence was the expeditious discharge of patients—patients who often had continuing postdischarge multiple health care needs. While attempting to control hospital costs, these regulations increased the need for health care that then had to be provided in the community. The second consequence was to effectively transfer the locus—where the majority of health is to be provided—from the hospital to the community.

Some evidence suggests that because patients were discharged "quicker and sicker," readmission rates and emergency room use increased, thus increasing the cost of health care (Dziegielewski, 1998). In fact, though controlling the annual rates of increase in the cost of health care, the DRGs were not successful in controlling total health care expenditures (Berkman, 1996). For instance, between 1984 and 1992, there was a 20 percent reduction in inpatient hospital days, an 11 percent reduction in the total number of hospital admissions, and a decrease in the annual rate of increase in health care costs (Shortell, Gillies, & Devers, 1995). However, total expenditures continued to increase; the total expenditure for health care in 1985 ($429 billion) more than doubled by 1995 ($989 billion) (Dziegielewski & Holliman, 2001).

Though total health care expenditures continued to rise under the DRGs, efforts to control the cost of health care persisted. By the mid-1990s, "managed care" systems were being implemented to extend cost control mechanisms beyond the hospital. Insurance providers, employers who offered insurance benefits to employees, and the government endeavored to constrain mounting health care expenditures and increase efficiency across the continuum of health care from inpatient to outpatient settings (Jenson, Morrisey, Gaffney, & Liston, 1997; Schneider, Hyer, & Luptak, 2000). Motivated by the increasing cost of health care and by a disarray of nationwide health care plans and reforms, managed care organizations developed to vertically and horizontally integrate services and funding coverage within competitive business- and market-based programs.

The dominance of managed care health care systems by the end of the 1990s, in the private sector and in Medicare and Medicaid, was evident. Though corporatized private management of health services had been slowly developing during the latter part of the twentieth century, by the end of the 1990s over four-fifths of patients were managed by twelve powerful managed care systems (Davidson, Davidson, & Keigher, 1999; Dziegielewski, 1998). A further indication of the rapid expansion of managed care organizations is the reported data that by the mid-1990s, nearly three-quarters (73 percent) of all outpatient visits billed to third party payers were under managed care systems (Berkman, 1996). More recently, data from 2001 suggest that 90 percent of workers with employer-sponsored health insurance are in some type of managed care system (Jensen & Morrisey, 2004). The expansion of managed care in health care coverage was not exclusive to private insurers. The number of Medicaid beneficiaries enrolled in some form of managed care increased from about 2 million in 1990 to nearly 12 million, or one-third of all beneficiaries, in 1995. By 2000, 40 percent of Medicaid recipients, of whom nearly all were women of childbearing age and children, were enrolled in a managed care plan (Weissman, Witzburg, Linov, & Campbell, 1999). It is expected that the proportion of children receiving Medicaid health benefits under managed care arrangements will continue to increase. However, because enrolling chronically ill or disabled children, whose health care is costly, is not advantageous to managed care organizations, these at-risk children may join the growing ranks of the uninsured (Deal & Shiono, 1998; Pear, 1999).

The growth and domination of managed care in health care in such a short span of time seems like an extremely rapid revolution. However, managed care has been around for some time, as a brief discussion of its history in the United States demonstrates.

A Brief History of Managing Health Care Delivery and Funding in the United States

Various types of systems to manage health care have existed in the United States since the early twentieth century. The roots of contemporary managed care programs may be traced to (1) early benevolent societies providing prepaid health care for immigrants and the poor and (2) benefit plans for the employees of large industries, such as lumber, railroads, and mining companies (Friedman, 1996). As an example of the former, the Benedictine Sisters in Minnesota, who organized and provided health care for the purchase of a health care "ticket," were early providers and managers of hospital and outpatient health care for the poor (Boo, 1991). In early employer/company-based health care programs, employees paid for benefits, and the company owned the hospitals and directly employed physicians. Examples of this era of managed health care are the Kaiser Permanente Health System (a California-based health system) and the Ford family-funded health care program of Detroit General Hospital, which provided physician-centered managed health care for employees and for the poor, respectively (Friedman, 1996). The first physician-hospital organization that paid capitation fees to physicians for providing health care to "members" (who paid $25 annually) was the Community Cooperative Hospital of Elk City, Oklahoma. The Cooperative, a prepaid program, was created and directed by a physician called Michael Shadid in 1931 in response to his frustration with the poor quality of health care and income-driven unnecessary surgeries (Shadid, 1959). The thread of benevolence is evident in these early efforts to offer and manage health care, unlike the overt business motivations of managed care systems currently (Starr, 1982, 1994).

Until the latter part of the twentieth century, organized and "managed" health care approaches were sporadic and idiosyncratic. Health maintenance organizations (HMOs) were developed initially by the employer-owners of large companies as "benefits" to workers. One such organization, the now familiar Kaiser Permanente Health System, was used by the lumber industries in Washington and California to recruit and retain employees (Cowles, 2003; Friedman, 1996). Since the mid-1970s, when public law legalized HMOs and expanded the definition of prepaid health care to include physicians in independent practice associations (Health Maintenance Organization Act of 1973, P.L. 93-222; Gorin, 2003), the number of HMOs in a variety of forms grew exponentially (Starr, 1994). A decade later, federal legislation, in an attempt to foster preventive and comprehensive care systems, created fiscal incentives for establishing for-profit managed care organizations to facilitate enrollment by Medicare and Medicaid recipients (Tax Equity and Fiscal Responsibility Act of 1982, P.L. 97-248). Multiple mergers and acquisitions resulted in the integration of systems into only a dozen mega–managed care organizations. By the mid-1990s, 85 percent of Americans who had health insurance were in some form of managed care (Davidson, Davidson, & Keigher, 1999).

To summarize, specific individuals and/or local/regional enterprises led the early ventures into the "managing" of health care. More recently, developments in managed health care resulted from a desire to compete more aggressively in the marketplace, to enhance profitability, and/or to control a specific market share, preferentially across the nation.

THE CHANGING STRUCTURE OF HEALTH CARE DELIVERY

The term "managed care" is not a single homogeneous construct, as managed care systems are complex and diverse. In general, managed care is a system for integrating health care delivery systems by approving the care rendered and also by following the patients throughout their care. Managed care is implemented through a variety of techniques that influence the provision of health care, health care consumers, and providers, and put in place administrative control of health care access, cost, and quality. In essence, managed care plans integrate the utilization (i.e., use of services), provision, and funding of health care (Dziegielewski & Holliman, 2001). Several techniques are used by managed care to control cost (Berkman, 1996; Dinerman, 1997; Redmond, 2001; Shortell & Hull, 1996). These include

- preauthorizing eligibility to receive specific care (i.e., precerting);
- predetermining the extent of care covered and provider fees;
- monitoring the type and extent of care provided;
- emphasizing health care delivery in outpatient, rather than inpatient, settings.

Although managed care plans are not uniform in how these techniques are specifically combined in the coverage plans, their overall objectives are clear and directly linked to cost control: to ensure that health care is provided with the most cost-effective treatments and interventions, said treatments and interventions are demonstrably effective, and all providers are accountable for the care that they render.

Theoretically, managed care seeks to assure adequate, quality health care with emphasis on prevention, while containing the cost of health care. Prevention of serious, and costly, illnesses, such as cancer and heart disease, is obviously important for the reduction of health care costs. It is informally, but widely, agreed that, in practice, managed care's top priority may not be quality comprehensive preventive health care, even though prevention strategies provided at the patient level of care are shown to be empirically effective (Amonkar, Madhavan, Rosenbluth, Odedina, & Simon, 2000).

Capitation, Efficiency, and Accountability

Managed care systems accomplish control of costs by endorsing those treatments that are the least costly and proven to be effective, by capitation payments to providers, and by making providers accountable for patient outcomes. These mechanisms control both what health providers do and patient utilization and, taken together, change the structure of how health care is delivered by inserting managed care systems into the process of delivering care at the level of providers and consumers.

Capitation is the hinge that holds the system of managed care together by imposing a fixed payment for a specific health care service or treatment. Capitation has some distinct advantages to health care providers and potential disadvantages to both patients and providers. One of the advantages to providers is that capitation assures them an expectable revenue stream. The fact that capitation is not adjustable when a patient's care requirements exceed the capitation fee is a disadvantage to providers and to patients (Schneider, Hyer, & Luptak, 2000).

Managed care organizations hold the provider accountable for both the effectiveness and efficiency of care, and for patient outcomes. Obviously, for a given patient, assuring that the services provided are not duplicative, overlapping, and/or conflicting is in the patient's best interests. Conversely, constraining care to the limits of a patient's managed care plan when that patient is in need of greater or more expensive care is not in the consumer's best interests. Before the dominance of managed care in health, and its insertion into the physician-patient relationship, the physician was the sole determiner of the type and duration of patient care. In contrast, managed care systems emphasize planning and implementation of health care services by interdisciplinary providers. Accordingly, interdisciplinary teamwork and decision making is gaining in importance. Nonetheless, the role of physicians now often includes being the agent, or "gatekeeper," for managed care systems governing patient access to all health services and prompting physicians to render the "least" care. This insertion of managed care systems as a "third party" to the traditional physician-patient relationship transformed the structure— the how and by whose authority—of delivering health care. To sum up, managed care controls costs by structurally controlling access to care, predetermining provider payments and the type of care, preventing duplication, holding providers accountable, and preferentially approving community-based rather than hospital/inpatient care.

THE CHANGING FOCUS
OF HEALTH CARE DELIVERY

The regulations and initiatives that attempted to control hospital care costs by limiting the duration of patients' hospitalizations changed the focus of health care from acute and episodic illnesses to chronic and predictable illnesses, and its structure from physician-centered to system controlled. Cost control is also achieved by limiting access to care, especially of high-cost patients. It has been suggested that the business priorities of managed health care organizations may motivate "cherry picking," or "creaming," of patients to assure that those patients who are at risk and needing expensive care, or who are without personal resources to pay for care, are not approved to receive care or whose care, if approved, is more diligently controlled (Feldman, 2001). Managed care organizations prefer healthy, low-risk consumers to those with complex health conditions, limited financial resources, and in need of costly medical care.

The focus on low-risk, less costly consumers is reinforced by the financial structure and the business philosophy of health care organizations. Currently, health care organizations—from managed care systems to hospitals and to providers—are increasingly for-profit corporatized systems or conglomerates, rather than nonprofit, autonomous, service-oriented providers and professionals. Consolidated health care systems are vertically and horizontally integrated and may include in one entity managed care organizations, nursing homes, pharmaceutical companies, hospitals, and provider groups (Gorin, 2003; Shortell & Hull, 1996). In some areas of the nation, all aspects of health care are managed, delivered, monitored, evaluated, and funded through a monopoly of one health care mega-corporation (Friedman, 1996). The business mindset of these organizations is to reward those who provide cost-effective care, rather than all the care a patient may need, and this stands in contrast to the prior fee-for-service compensation systems that financially rewarded for providing more, rather than less, care.

To put it concisely, the overall emphasis on cost vigilance of managed care organizations transformed where, how, what type, and for whom health care is delivered. The changes in health care resulting from the revolution in funding include a shift in

- the locus of health care delivery from institutional to community care settings;
- the structure of health care delivery from the centrality of the physician's role to the centrality of the managed care system.

Types of Managed Care Systems

In order to understand managed care fully, some familiarity with the main types of programs is constructive. These are HMOs, preferred provider organizations (PPOs), point of service (POS) plans, and exclusive provider organizations (EPOs).

For many, HMOs are the sin qua non for "managed care." These cover services for members by integrating both health care insurance and health care delivery in one plan based on prepaid member fees/premiums. Services from outside the HMO "network" of providers is covered only at the discretion of the HMO. Some HMOs directly employ individual physicians, others employ multiple-physician groups, and still others employ a network of physicians to provide care for HMO members.

- PPOs cover services at a predetermined rate for its members through a network of providers, and generally do not cover services obtained out of the network of providers.
- POS plans, the most flexible of managed care models, have a group of approved providers, but do not preclude members from receiving care outside that system with comparatively minimal out of pocket costs to the patient.
- EPOs, the most restrictive type of managed care plans, cover only care delivered by approved providers and care provided out of this network is not eligible for coverage.

Last, pervasive cost vigilance across private and government coverage plans and programs realigned the focus of health care to preferentially serving healthy, low-risk patient populations. It is noteworthy that the focus on healthy, low-risk consumers seems contrary to one consequence of reducing hospital care—the increasing population with ongoing, complex health care needs. The latter topic is discussed in Chapter 2 on health consumer populations.

CHANGES IN GOVERNMENT FUNDING FOR FAITH-BASED ORGANIZATIONS AND WELFARE

Recent health care funding changes extend beyond the umbrella of managed care. Two particular comparatively recent changes in government funding are relevant to social work in community-based health care: (1) funding for faith-based organizations (FBOs) and (2) the health-related components of welfare reform legislation.

Government Funding for FBOs

By the late 1990s regulations for government funding for nonprofit organizations, with specific mention of FBOs, underwent significant changes (Chambre, 2001; Cnaan & Boddie, 2002). Charitable Choice legislation may level the playing field between secular and nonsecular service providers who compete for public funding. A section of the Federal Welfare Reform Act of 1996 established new, and for some, radical policies concerning the relationship of government funding and FBOs. This legislation and the Charitable Choice Expansion Act of 1999 prohibit public officials from discriminating against FBOs in competing for government-funded grants and contracts. Not only are FBOs protected against discrimination in government funding, but also as funding recipients, FBOs are granted the rights

- to retain authority over their mission and boards;
- to maintain a religious atmosphere in their agencies;
- to hire staff who agree with the religious beliefs.

In 2001, the White House Office of Faith-Based and Community Initiatives was implemented by executive order to increase FBO services and programs. Several individual states have instituted mechanisms to facilitate funding while others have implemented legislation to protect religious freedom (Cnaan & Boddie, 2002; The White House, 2003).

These funding legislative and executive orders both promote funding opportunities for FBOs and limit their use of those funds. The regulations prohibit FBOs from using government funds for sectarian worship, religious instruction, or proselytizing consumers. In addition, an FBO receiving government funding cannot treat the consumers differently on the basis of their religion or faith, or their refusal to participate in particular religious activities. The types of relationships between government-funding entities and FBOs include direct funding, indirect funding, and nonfinancial arrangements. Indirect funding occurs between government funding agencies and an intermediary subcontracted FBO, such as Goodwill Industries. Nonfinancial collaborations include arrangements where the government provides in-kind, nonmonetary assistance, such as office space or use of vehicles, or when FBOs provide services for clients referred to them by local welfare agencies.

According to recent research, faith-based funding legislation appears to have resulted in faith-based programs developing services for the working poor, as well as the unemployed or welfare dependent, and expanding existing services and programs beyond their traditional focus on concrete services. Recent efforts by FBOs include face-to-face psychosocial and counseling services, and health care and health-related programs (Hodge & Pittman, 2003; Sherman, 2000). Cnaan and Boddie (2002) suggest that as a corollary to Charitable Choice legislation and funding availability, more FBOs are providing social and health care services based on congregational, rather than government, funding. These latter developments may reflect concerns on the part of some FBOs regarding the Charitable Choice legislation restrictions, as discussed previously, or reluctance to engaging in processes that include governmental oversight.

Changes in the Health Care Coverage in Welfare Programs

Welfare reform legislation in the 1990s changed Medicaid health care benefits by limiting both the amount and duration of benefits, and by restricting the eligibility criteria. The Personal Responsibility and Work Reconciliation Act of 1996 (P.L. 104-193) disconnected the previous automatic link between cash receipt of welfare and health care coverage. The individual states retain discretion in extending coverage beyond the limits of the act. However, research findings suggest that significantly more of those terminated from Medicaid coverage as a result of the legislation have reduced access to health care, cannot get needed prescription drugs, go without needed health care, and experience poorer health than either those remaining on Medicaid or those with private insurance (Weissman, Witzburg, Linov, & Campbell, 1999). It is possible that reforms to reduce the number of Americans economically dependent on welfare merely resulted in increases in the number of uninsured people (Pear, 1999). In an attempt to maintain health care coverage for poor children who, because of these welfare reforms, are not eligible for Medicaid health care coverage, the Balanced Budget Act of 1997 created funding for their health care coverage in the form of the Child Health Insurance Program (CHIP). However, this legislation, and incremental efforts by states, has done little to prevent the expansion of the uninsured/underinsured population. The population of uninsured/underinsured Americans is discussed in Chapter 2.

In conclusion, funding for health care underwent multiple incremental changes in philosophical underpinnings, policies, and regulations including several iterations of funding reforms and the dominance of managed care principles and organizations. The result is a health care system that prioritizes

- cost containment;
- accountability;
- care provided outside hospitals and institutions;
- healthier, and therefore, lower cost consumers.

These priorities realign the relationship of providers and consumers, replacing the authority of the physician with the authority of a third party that preapproves, monitors, and evaluates the care provided. Recent evidence suggests that managed care has not been effective in controlling costs and that interim reductions in national health care costs are the result of cost-shifting by raising the insured portion of premiums, deductibles, and copayments and the escalating costs associated with advances in medical technology (Clemmitt, 2001; Gorin, 2003; Strunk & Ginsburg, 2004).

ETHICAL CONSIDERATIONS

Managed care is pervasive in health care with every likelihood of being here to stay. Because of managed care principles and programs that constrain coverage and health care resource use, ethical dilemmas for social workers can occur. For example, when the social worker must choose between two or more relevant, but opposing, ethical obligations or when every alternative results in an undesirable outcome for one or more persons (Lowenberg, Dolgoff, & Harrington, 2000). A practitioner can experience an ethical conflict when faced by two or more competing professional values, such as the well-being of the client and of the agency.

There are many ethical considerations and dilemmas in social work practice in community health care centers, such as between financial and administrative priorities of managed care and other funding systems and the influence of those priorities on health care agencies, organizations, and health care consumers (Kane, Houston-Vega, & Nuehring, 2002; Reamer, 1997; Rock & Congress, 1999). Specifically, these potentially competing interests may result in conflicts concerning the ethical obligation of practitioners to consumers to assure consumer well-being and consumer confidentiality, and to their employing agency and its well-being. Revisions to the NASW's *Code of Ethics* (2001) include ethical obligations to

- disclose confidential information to third parties only with client authorization;
- ensure the security and confidentiality of written and electronic records (including telephones, computers, facsimile, telephone answering systems, and so on);
- attend to their employing organizations' financial needs while not permitting organizational or administrative policies or procedures to interfere with ethical practice with clients.

To resolve ethical conflicts between the financial and limited service priorities of managed care, social workers are required to be skilled in analyzing their ethical obligations to both the well-being of their employing organization and the biopsychosocial well-being of their clients.

Analyzing these ethical conflicts is only the first step, however. Once analyzed, resolving these dilemmas requires skills in effective advocacy on behalf of consumers with managed care entities and with agency administrators and colleagues from non–social work disciplines. Given the emphasis on cost-effectiveness and limited resource utilization of managed care, and the needs of agencies to maintain managed care revenues, cost-benefit, and cost-effectiveness, there is value-added empirical evidence substantiating the fact that needed psychosocial interventions beneficial to the agency, the managed care organization, and the consumer are indispensable.

Social workers' ethical obligation to ensure health care consumer well-being is not superceded by decisions of managed care systems to limit care. Under these circumstances, practitioners are obligated not only to advocate for the consumer, but also to take steps to prevent client abandonment and assure that clients receive needed services. Terminating services and referral to other providers cannot rest on depleted benefits, limited coverage for care, or managed care rationing of resources (Reamer, 1997). Though social workers may be pressured to comply with the limitation of care priorities of managed care, practitioners must be prepared to offer pro bono services and to advocate for doing so with their agencies. In these circumstances, careful, thorough, and well-documented efforts, including discussions with consumers concerning termination and referral, must occur to assure that the needs of the clients for ongoing care are met with timely and quality services.

The documentation requirements of managed care and the use of computer technology for transfer of client information present yet another area of potential ethical dilemmas over consumers' confidentiality versus disclosure. Client confidentiality is fundamental to an effective worker-client relationship and a core social work value. However, consumer confidentiality in the environment of managed care third parties is not absolute, but relative, or qualified, due to the necessity of transferring confidential consumer information to third parties to substantiate the need for services, and to document services provided and patient outcomes (Gelman, Pollack, & Weiner, 1999).

Rock and Congress (1999) specify the requirements of social workers concerning consumer confidentiality in relation to managed care systems. Requirements include

- fully informed and documented consumer consent including what information will need to be transferred to managed care organizations;
- specific limits of confidentiality concerning disclosure of child abuse and potential harm to the consumer or others.

In addition, managed care systems require social workers to include documentation of the type, duration, and payment arrangements of services, and that consumers understand and agree to the transfer of this information in written informed consent forms (Kane, Houston-Vega, & Nuehring, 2002).

Consumer confidentiality and the use of technology to transfer consumer information, including access to and the security of these computer systems, is an area of growing concern. Technological transfer of client information includes land lines, cell phones, and fax in addition to computers, e-mail, and computer databases. The legal obligations and requirements of HIPAA (Health Insurance Portability and Accountability Act of 1996, P.L. 104-191), implemented in 2003, are specific regarding the transfer of and access to individually identifiable consumer health data through any venue (Callaway & Venegas, 2003). The intent of the privacy rules of HIPAA is to protect consumers' rights over access to and the use of their health information and to assure the security of medical records. Although the privacy components of HIPAA were implemented in 2003, the security provisions for these components await implementation.

HIPAA covers all those who provide, bill, or pay for medical care and those who process health consumer information (i.e., health care clearinghouses). A health care provider is defined as anyone who furnishes health care, bills for, or is paid for care provided; social workers are included as health providers. Health plans include all government organizations, private organizations, and individuals that provide for, process information, or pay medical costs. Last, health care clearinghouses—organizations that receive health information from providers and manage or transform that information for claims—include those that provide billing services and third party administration. Health information (i.e., protected health information or PHI) is specifically defined to include any information, whether spoken, electronic, or written, that refers to the health of an individual or to the payment for care provided and that could directly or indirectly be used to identify that individual. Individual health information (IHI) includes age, geographic information, zip code, gender, race, ethnicity, and marital status. The issue is, of course, disclosure and confidentiality. Specifically, HIPAA requires that no information be transferred through any medium unless the consumer, or his or her legally specified agent, approves in writing that transmittal, unless otherwise permitted or required by law, and that any transmittal be only the minimum necessary information.

The regulations detail what must be included in consent forms, including certain diseases of public health concern, child abuse, elder abuse, neglect, and domestic violence. HIPAA also requires consumer authorization for the release of information that specifies what and to whom. Social workers in community health must be knowledgeable of HIPAA regulations, receive the required training, and be cognizant of how the regulations both protect consumer confidentiality and where that confidentiality may be vulnerable to the administrative practices and computer system and technologies, and day-to-day procedures utilized in their community health settings. Notably, the NASW, in its revision of the profession's *Code of Ethics* (2001), included social workers' ethical obligations to inform all clients of the types of information and to be diligent concerning the security of client information in all paper and electronic forms as detailed by HIPAA.

Briefly, ethical practice in community-based health care can only be provided by social workers that are knowledgeable about state and federal laws concerning confidentiality and its limits, the NASW *Code of Ethics,* managed care regulations and their agencies' computer technology, voice mail, paging, instant messaging, and computer/database security systems.

THE INFLUENCES OF MANAGED CARE ON PRACTICE

Social workers practicing in the current environment of managed health care—especially with vulnerable, at-risk populations of consumers—need to be competent in several areas of practice. The cost vigilance and accountability emphases of managed care and other third parties on gatekeeping and evidence-based interventions are here to stay. In order to meet that mandate, social workers must understand not only the pragmatic business principles of the new health paradigm, but also how these priorities impact social work practice in community-based health care settings, effective interdisciplinary collaboration, leadership, and documentation skills that are critically important in this environment. Practitioners in community health need to be competent in consumer, program, and population level practice, and in practice and program evaluation (Berkman & Maramaldi, 2001; Kane, Houston-Vega, & Nuehring, 2002; Lesser, 2000; Rosenberg,

1998; Schneider, Hyer, & Luptak, 2000; Volland, Berkman, Phillips, & Stein, 2003).

Specifically, the knowledge and skills for practice necessitated by managed care and the revolution in health care funding include

- the goals, policies, and expectations of a variety of health care funding plans, policies, and programs, including government, managed care, and reduced fee resources;
- time-saving and cost-efficient evidence-based assessment tools, screening instruments, and interventions;
- developing and evaluating consumer outcomes and translating the findings in terms of practice- and cost-effectiveness;
- collaborative interdisciplinary practice;
- documentation requirements.

Opportunities in Social Work Practice in Community-Based Health Care

The revolution in funding transformed the locus, the structure, and the focus of health care delivery. These transformations, the prevalence of managed care, and the corporatization of health care create opportunities for social workers in community-based health care settings. For example, opportunities are emerging in

- innovative programs to deliver health care through new venues, particularly to vulnerable populations;
- community prevention;
- leadership in community, interorganizational, and interdisciplinary programs;
- primary care settings.

Primary care is a setting in ambulatory health care that is growing in response to the mandates of managed care for the designation of a primary provider for patients. Not surprisingly, social work in primary care settings is also growing as a field of practice for reasons related to the priorities of managed care making primary physicians rely more on social workers for three reasons (Lesser, 2000). Primary care is endorsed by managed care systems; empirical evidence supports the relation of medical conditions, psychosocial issues, and behavioral issues; and physicians have limited time for direct patient care and psychosocial content in medical education is scarce (Zayas & Dyche, 1992). In sum, these factors may increase physicians' receptivity to collaboration with social workers in primary care settings.

Opportunities for social workers are also expanding in innovative programs for vulnerable and at-risk populations that integrate multiple disciplines and service providers in one setting. As an illustration, integrated interdisciplinary, collaborative health centers can include in one location providers from public health departments and clinics, hospitals, social welfare programs, mental health institutions, community colleges, police, juvenile justice departments, community resources, churches, and educational institutions (U.S. Department of Health and Human Services, 1999; Pecukonis, Cornelius, & Parrish, 2003; Powell et al., 2001).

In brief, social workers in community-based health care who are knowledgeable about the complexities of funding, managed care systems, and sources for the under- and uninsured consumer can assist the consumer's journey across increasingly complex health care systems. Advocacy skills at all levels of practice are essential in the cost-sensitive arena of health care, as are skills in documentation substantiating consumer needs for service and health outcomes. Skills in resolving ethical conflicts due to information technology, third party access to client information, and related legalities are central to practice in community health. The value of the knowledge and skill to demonstrate the benefit as well as the effectiveness of social work cannot be overstated.

SUMMARY

In conclusion, this chapter explored the influences leading to the revolution in funding; the history of health care delivery and management in the United States; the priorities, principles, and mechanisms of managed care; and funding changes for FBOs and welfare recipients. A discussion of social work ethical considerations in light of these topics identified the conflicts potentiated by limitations in care and coverage, the technological transfer of client information, and HIPAA regulations. The chapter concluded with a discussion of social work practice in ambulatory health in view of the influences of the shifts in the locus, structure, and focus of health care delivery.

DISCUSSION QUESTIONS AND ACTIVITIES FOR INDIVIDUALS AND SMALL GROUPS

1. Engage in conversations with non–social work health care professionals, such as physicians, nurses, and physical therapists, regarding their professional and personal view of managed care. You might consider having one or more such professionals address the class. Questions to explore: How do different disciplines see the role of managed care? How do different disciplines view the disparate access of some populations of health consumers?
2. Compare the responses to question 1 to the responses of fellow social workers: What do you think underlie the varying disciplinary views and responses? How are professional values of each discipline evidenced in their views?

GLOSSARY

advocacy: Practice activities including educating, informing, or presenting the needs of individual and family consumers, or on behalf of groups or populations of consumers.

capitation: One technique of managed care to control costs by setting a fixed monetary amount(s) paid prospectively to health care providers per patient for a health care service or treatment regardless of the cost of that services.

cherry picking/creaming: A process used by managed care and/or organizations to deliberately select consumers who are the healthiest and have insurance coverage over consumers with complex, multiple health and psychosocial problems, or consumers who are frail and underresourced.

DRGs: Diagnosis related groups; a system whose regulations were implemented in the mid-1980s to reduce the lengths of hospitalizations and predetermine coverage for a given specific medical diagnosis.

EPOs: Exclusive provider organizations; a type of HMO plan.

for-profit/proprietary organizations: The primary goal these organizations is to yield profit from revenues; may have nonprofit divisions or subsidiary sections of the organization; primary funding through fees for services.

health care consumers: Individuals who utilize health care and health care–related services; depending on the setting may be referred to as clients (e.g., social service clients), participants (e.g., community program participants), and/or patients (medical or mental health patients).

health care providers: According to HIPAA all those who supply health care and associated services and manage, organize, or compile consumer health information.

HMOs: Health maintenance organizations; a term used to generally identify managed care systems.

LOS: Length of stay; duration of a patient's stay for a single inpatient hospitalization; generally designated as a specific number of days.

managed care: A variety of techniques utilized to influence providers and patients by integrating payment and delivery of health care; goal is to balance quantity and quality of time-limited health care services while maintaining cost-efficiency.

Medicaid: A federal and state government funded program that provides payment for the medical care of persons who meet certain means-tested criteria.

Medicare: A federal government medical insurance program under the Social Security Act that funds the medical care of Social Security beneficiaries.

nonprofit organizations: Organizations that provide services or programs representing the interests of a community or group whose revenues must support the organizations' programs and services, rather than profits; primary funding through charitable contribution, but may also receive governmental funding.

POS: Point of service; a type of HMO plan.

PPOs: Preferred provider organizations; a type of HMO plan.

public organizations: Organizations that receive funding through allocation of tax dollars to provide human services.

Chapter 2

The Health Care
Consumer Population

- *How are longevity and diversification changing the consumer population?*
- *What is chronic illness? Why is the population of the chronically ill growing?*
- *What are the major chronic illnesses and risk factors that are associated with cultural diversity?*
- *Who are the uninsured/underinsured and how do they get health care?*
- *How are psychosocial and behavioral characteristics and illnesses linked?*

INTRODUCTION

Several trends are changing the demographic characteristics and care needs of the health care consumer population in the United States. These trends are the increasing number and proportions of the health care consumer population who (1) are living longer; (2) are racially and culturally diverse; (3) have chronic illnesses; (4) are underinsured or uninsured; (5) have or are at risk for specific illnesses; and/or (6) have medical conditions closely associated with

Social Work Practice in Community-Based Health Care
© 2007 by The Haworth Press, Inc. All rights reserved.
doi:10.1300/5273_02

psychosocial characteristics or behaviors. These changes in the health consumer population require that social workers in ambulatory health

- understand each of these changes;
- understand how these changes interact to create risk factors and vulnerabilities in the health care consumer population;
- have basic knowledge of the major health conditions of the health care consumer population overall, and particularly of at-risk health care consumer populations.

Healthy People 2010 is the federal government plan that identifies a comprehensive list of prevention and health promotion objectives for the nation. The two major goals are (1) to increase the quality and years of healthy life and (2) to eliminate health disparities. Under these two major goals, the Healthy People 2010 plan identifies twenty-eight focus areas, such as access to quality health care, diabetes, heart disease and stroke, educational and community-based programs, HIV (human immunodeficiency virus), and maternal, infant, and child health (Centers for Disease Control, 2003b; U.S. Department of Health and Human Services, 2002).

In summary, the factors influencing the health consumer population noted earlier and the goals and focus areas of Healthy People 2010 shape both social work practice in community-based health care and the content of this chapter. This chapter explores each of the areas noted in relation to social work practice in community-based health care.

INCREASING LONGEVITY

Increasing longevity—living longer—is a benefit of better health care overall and advances in medicine during the latter decades of the twentieth century. Increased longevity suggests the likelihood of extending an individual's lifespan and, collectively, increases the number of persons in the population living longer (U.S. Census Bureau, 2000b). For example, by 2025 the average lifespan in the United States will be eighty-two years for women and seventy-six years for men (Pecukonis, Cornelius, & Parrish, 2003). As a result of the aging of the "Baby Boom" generation (i.e., those 75 million persons born in the United States between 1946 and 1964) and advances in medicine and medical technologies, the number of persons aged sixty-five and older is projected to double by the middle of the century (Hobbs & Damon, 1996). It is estimated that by midcentury, one-third of Americans will be over sixty-five years of age, nearly triple the proportion of those sixty-five years of age in the population in 1990 (i.e., 13 percent) (Dhooper, 2003; Sudha & Multran, 2001). We have come to accept on some level that the society in which we live is an aging society. However, in terms of the impact on our health care systems and consumers, we have not articulated that acceptance into a health care delivery system that can provide care to health care consumers across the lifespan in the magnitude projected.

To sum up, the expansion of the aging population and overall increasing longevity combined with the shift to community-based health care require health care social workers in community-based practice who understand health disparities, chronic illness, and their impact on the daily lives, and the physical and psychosocial health care needs of consumers across the lifespan.

THE DIVERSIFICATION OF HEALTH CARE CONSUMERS

The increasing diversity of the U.S. population is the result of the increasing pace of immigration over the last decades of the twentieth century. Of all immigrants in the United States, 60 percent arrived since 1980 and 20 percent arrived since 1990 (Keigher, 1997). The immigrant population is now also much more heterogeneous than in previous decades as is the population overall. In the census of 2000, 2.4 percent reported they were of two or more races (U.S. Census Bureau, 2004).

In relation to health care, recent legislation, such as the Personal Responsibility and Work Opportunity Act (1996), targeted immigrants in its restrictions to resources, set employment as an eligibility requirement for welfare assistance, and delayed eligibility for five years after immigration (Cornelius, 2000). As a result, those who immigrate to America in this century may be particularly at risk for limited, restricted access to care and to poor health.

It is estimated that the Hispanic and Asian populations in the United States will triple by 2050. Projections suggest that Hispanic Americans will make up nearly one-quarter of the population, or 103 million persons, and Asian Americans will constitute 8 percent of the population, or 33 million individuals (CNN News, 2004). The number of African Americans will increase from 36 million to 61 million, or 14.6 percent of the population, whereas, conversely, the non-Hispanic white population is decreasing and estimated to be less than one-half of the population by the middle of this century, and women will continue to outnumber men (U.S. Census Bureau, 2000).

The older population also reflects the rapid diversification of the U.S. population. For example, in the 1990 census, less than 4 percent of older adults were Hispanic; by 2050, that proportion is expected to more than triple (i.e., 15.5 percent) (U.S. Census Bureau, 2004). Overall, in the 1990s, minorities were 13 percent of older adults; by 2020, 23 percent of elders will be of minority groups (Pinquart & Sorensen, 2005).

Interactions of Race, Economic Status, Gender, and Health

Health status varies by race, economic status, and gender (Institute of Medicine, 2002). Morbidity rates—the rates of persons who are limited in their daily activities, often referred to as "instrumental" activities, such as activities at work, shopping, or household tasks, due to chronic conditions—are higher for minority populations and for women compared to men. By way of illustration, a higher proportion of African (14.3 percent), than of white, non-Hispanic Americans (11.5 percent) report that they experience some limitation in daily activities due to chronic health conditions (Appel, Harrell, & Deng, 2002). Appel et al. also report that while cardiovascular disease (CVD) is the leading overall cause of death in the United States, the rates of morbidity and of mortality due to CVD are greater for African Americans than non-Hispanic white Americans. More minorities reported that their health is fair or poor than do white, non-Hispanic populations (Centers for Disease Control, 2002a).

Interacting with these health disparities by racial category is the consistent correlation between poverty and poor health. More Americans living at or below the poverty threshold report fair or poor health than in the nonpoor population (20.9 percent versus 6.3 percent, respectively) (U.S. Office of Women's Health, 2004). Overall, infants of minority populations have mortality rates that are 2.5 times higher than white, non-Hispanic infants. For example, infant mortality rates for African Americans and for Native Americans is more than 1.5 times that of non-Hispanic whites. Disparities in income may explain disparities in health status; over one-quarter of African Americans, but less than one-tenth of non-Hispanic white Americans, live below the poverty line (Appel, Harrell, & Deng, 2002). Notably, both African Americans and Native American populations are also disproportionately unemployed and undereducated.

Race and gender interact in health disparities as well. As an illustration, while African Americans overall have greater rates of CVD than whites, African-American women have greater rates of stroke, less improvement in mortality rates from CVD, and overall shorter life expectancies than both African-American men and all non-Hispanic white Americans (American Heart Association 2004). More women of African-American and Hispanic populations (20 and 29 percent respectively) report they are in fair or poor health than do white women (13 percent); the rate of hypertension among African-American women (57 percent) is twice that of non-Hispanic white women (28 percent) (Kaiser Family Foundation, 2004).

Morbidity rates also vary disproportionately by race and gender. A higher proportion of African Americans (19.2 percent) report needing help in their daily activities, such as household chores, because of chronic health conditions than do non-Hispanic white (12.1 percent) women (U.S. Office of Women's Health, 2004).

Briefly, the health care consumer population reflects the aging and diversification of the overall population in the United States. The health status of minority populations is poorer and their disability rates are higher than in the white population. Poverty, racial category, and gender consistently interact in relation to poor health indicators and rates of disability. These interactions mean that a large, and growing, proportion of the health care consumer population in the United States is at risk for poor health; disproportionate rates of morbidity, mortality, and disability; and chronic illness.

CHRONIC ILLNESS

Chronic physical illness is defined as a serious, ongoing health condition that has a biological, anatomical, or physiologic basis and has lasted, or is expected to last, at least one year. In addition, for an illness to be defined as chronic, it either must produce or, in relation to "expectable-normal" functioning, is likely to produce one or more of the following:

- shortened life expectancy;
- disability;
- disfigurement;
- limitation(s) of function or activities;
- necessity for surgical intervention;
- requirement for ongoing medical treatments;
- dependency on medication and/or special diets;
- dependency on medical technology.

For consumers, and their families, normative initial reactions to having a chronic illness, or of receiving a diagnosis of a chronic illness, include an acute sense of helplessness (feeling overwhelmed), a sense of loss stemming from the loss of previously anticipated abilities and wellness, fear of the unknown, and/or anger. Several mediating factors may ease or deter adjustment to living with a chronic illness. These include the life stage of the consumer at the time of the onset of the chronic illness, gender (i.e., in general women tend to successfully adjust better than men), whether the illness is socially stigmatized (e.g., HIV+/AIDS), race/ethnicity, the degree of uncertainty in the disease course, and family relationships (Widerman, 2004).

Factors Increasing the Population of the Chronically Ill

Advances in medicine, medical technology, and increasing longevity have increased the number of consumers who are chronically ill. The proportion of the population with chronic illnesses is expected to increase rapidly and continuously. By the end of the present decade, the proportion of the population who are chronically ill is expected to reach 14 percent (Pecukonis, Cornelius, & Parrish, 2003).

Technological and medical advances dramatically transform once terminal and acute illnesses into chronic conditions. As a specific illustration, advances in the treatment for childhood cancers, such as several childhood leukemias, have greatly improved the cure rates over recent years (Zebrack & Chesler, 2000). The number of survivors of pediatric cancer—who may have lifelong health care and psychosocial needs because of having cancer, surviving cancer, and having received extensive cancer treatments—expands annually due to improvements in medical treatments. Lifelong psychosocial needs, according to the research findings of Zebrack and Chesler (2000, 2001), include worries over a recurrence of cancer, their own children having cancer, and general health worries; women tended to have more worries than men. As the researchers note, the ongoing, long-term psychosocial and supportive services to address these needs are often sporadic and inconsistent.

A second example of the transformation of another once catastrophic disease to a long-term condition is AIDS—acquired immunodeficiency syndrome—caused by an HIV infection. The length of time from diagnosis to death from AIDS was once quite short. Through extensive pharmaceutical research, there are now medicines available that stabilize HIV infection and the progression of AIDS, transforming the previously acute and fatal development of AIDS into a long-term chronic condition (Bontempi, Burleson, & Lopez, 2004; Mitchell & Linsk, 2004). Living successfully with an HIV infection is associated with multiple psychosocial challenges and health care needs requiring ongoing, community-based health and psychosocial care.

Technological advances in medicine are also changing once terminal traumatic injuries to long-term conditions. For example, brain and spinal cord trauma were once fatal or resulted in irreversible extensive paralysis. During the last decade, the outcomes of brain and spinal cord trauma underwent a transformation due to advances in emergency and posttrauma technologies (Degeneffe, 2001). Nonetheless, of the 1.5 million to 2 million Americans who experience traumatic brain injuries (TBI) each year, between 70 thousand and 90 thousand have long-term functional impairments requiring twenty-four-hour care; several hundred thousand more require less intense, but nonetheless, lifelong health care. The effects of TBI and spinal cord injuries are extensive including problems with cognition, memory, and problem solving; seizures; paralysis; sensory impairments; mobility; and personality and behavioral changes. A trauma survivor's family provides the majority of all care, with reported higher levels of stress and greater physical, psychosocial, and emotional needs than noncaregivers (Degeneffe, 2001; Rivera, Shewchuk, & Elliott, 2003).

Both survivors and their caregivers need ongoing psychosocial, in addition to medical, services and care—those social workers are skilled in providing.

Major Medical Conditions and Diverse Consumer Populations

Three medical conditions that are affecting large and increasing numbers of Americans, particularly in diverse populations, are diabetes, pediatric asthma, and HIV infection. Interestingly, but perhaps not surprisingly, the etiology of these three medical conditions is associated with limited access to health care and social and economic disadvantage. Predictable as it might be in a racialized society such as ours, health statistics and epidemiology data are collected, analyzed, and reported by racial category, as depicted in Table 2.1.

These four health conditions are more widespread and pose risk factors for culturally diverse populations, who also, due to the recent changes in health care funding discussed in Chapter 1, are less likely to have health care coverage and access. Because social workers in community-based health care need basic knowledge of major illnesses, the following sections discuss each condition in some detail.

Diabetes

Diabetes is the sixth leading cause of death in the United States (U.S. Department of Health and Human Services, 2001). Overall, 5.9 percent of the population is diabetic; the prevalence rate is increasing in the general population, and particularly among minority groups. The overall rate of diabetes in the adult population (type 2) increased from 4.9 percent to 6.5 percent from 1990 to 1998 (U.S. Department of Health and Human Services, 2001).

TABLE 2.1. Three major chronic illnesses by racial category.

Racial category	Diabetes[a] (≥ 20 years of age) (%)	Pediatric asthma[b] (<18 years of age) (%)	HIV+[c]
Hispanic	8.2	10.30	13,069
Asian American, Native Hawaiian, and Pacific Islander		10.60	644
Non-Hispanic Black	11.4	17.70	74, 988
Alaskan Native and American Indian	14.9	15.30	830
Non-Hispanic White	8.4	11.00	53,145

[a]U.S. Department of Health and Human Services, 2001; Diabetes rates among Asian Americans, Native Hawaiians, and Pacific Islanders are not available.

[b]American Lung Association, 2003.

[c]Centers for Disease Control, 2003a; HIV numbers are incidence numbers (i.e., the number of new cases) for the calendar year 2002 with all ages included rather than population estimates (i.e., prevalence) due to the confidentiality of HIV information.

As can be seen in Table 2.1, African Americans, Alaskan Natives, and American Indians have higher prevalence rates for diabetes than non-Hispanic whites. African Americans are between 1.4 and 2.2 times and American Indians 2.8 times more likely to have diabetes than non-Hispanic whites (U.S. Department of Health and Human Services, 2001). Rates of diabetes also differ by gender. The rate of diabetes (type 2) for adult African-American women (25 percent) is nearly twice, and a mortality rate 40 percent higher, than that of white women (Auslander, Haire-Joshu, Houston, Rhee, & Williams, 2002).

Diabetes is a disorder of the body's ability to utilize glucose (i.e., sugar) in the blood resulting in inadequate control of sugar levels by insulin. When glucose builds up in the blood instead of going into cells, the cells are starved for nutrients and other body systems have to provide energy for bodily functions. Diabetes is caused by the inability of the insulin-producing cells of the pancreas to produce enough insulin or to an inadequate response of the body's cells to the action of insulin, or a combination of these factors. Insufficient insulin or insufficient utilization of insulin prevents glucose from moving into cells resulting in increased glucose levels. Uncontrolled diabetes has many long-term and potentially life-threatening sequelae (U.S. Department of Health and Human Services, 2001). These are

- dehydration;
- weight loss;
- retinal damage leading to blindness;
- severe skin ulcerations;
- amputations resulting from impaired circulation, kidney damage, coma, and death;
- hardening of the arteries;
- heart disease;
- hypertension.

Type 1 diabetes, whose onset is generally in childhood, historically was also referred to as juvenile diabetes. Normally, the body's immune system fights off foreign invaders like viruses or bacteria. In type 1 diabetes, however, the immune system attacks insulin-producing cells resulting in a deficiency of insulin production. Type 2 diabetes, often called non-insulin-dependent diabetes, is the most common form of diabetes, affecting 18.2 million Americans, most of whom are adults. The causality of type 2 diabetes is more complex than that of type 1; here the body produces sufficient insulin, but the cells are resistant to the actions of insulin.

Complications from diabetes include end-stage renal disease requiring lifelong renal dialysis, heart disease, and retinal damage that can lead to irreversible blindness. Complication rates differ by population group. For instance, diabetics across all minority groups are at greater risk for early state kidney disease resulting from diabetes than white diabetics (Centers for Disease Control, 2003b). Some of these differing rates of complications are dramatic (American Diabetes Association, 2005). For example,

- the prevalence rate of retinal damage among Hispanic diabetics is 32-40 percent;
- amputation of lower limbs for First Nations peoples with diabetes is 3-4 times more likely than the general population of diabetics;
- Mexican-American diabetics are 6.6 times more likely to have end-stage renal disease than other diabetic populations.

It is likely that the social causes underlying these varying rates are related to differential access to health care, the health effects of poverty, perhaps culturally linked health beliefs about diabetes, and/or nutrition (Philis-Tsimikas & Walker, 2001).

Diabetes is costly for society owing to related increased costs of disability, mortality, and health care. Health care costs for patients with diabetes, largely due to more frequent and extensive care for cardiovascular complications, are more than four times greater than for similar patients without diabetes (Bertera, 2003). Diabetes also poses a heavy psychosocial and lifestyle burden on persons with diabetes and their families.

The psychosocial impact on the individual and his or her family is related to the age of the diabetic at the time of diagnosis and to the diabetic treatment required across the lifespan. The treatment for either type of diabetes usually includes nutritional regimens and/or medication, either in oral or injectable form, to gain effective control of blood sugar levels and thus prevent the negative sequelae associated with the disease. Clearly, these treatments require changes in lifestyle and behaviors. For children and teens, in the throes of adolescent psychosocial and physical development, adhering to strict dietary and medication schedules is difficult. The families of diabetic youths are wholly responsible for their teens' daily adherence to the dietary, medication, and exercise requirements of diabetic regimens (Bertera, 2003). Families must cope with the stress of the developmental and psychosocial needs, and the chronic illness of their children and teens.

Cultural background and related health beliefs regarding nutrition, eating rituals, alternative health therapies, and the spiritually based beliefs about individual responsibility for health are found to influence dietary and medication adherence, and effective control of diabetes (DeCoster, 2003; DeCoster & Cummings, 2004). For example, the significantly higher rate of diabetes in African Americans is linked to the greater amount of fat in their traditional diet compared to non-Hispanic whites, even after controlling for other risk factors (Auslander, Haire-Joshu, Houston, Rhee, & Williams, 2002). Minority populations of persons with diabetes have significantly higher rates of complications, including vision loss, amputations, and renal disease, and more difficulty in gaining control over the condition than non-Hispanic whites (Bertera, 2003).

Research on the relationship of family structure and diabetes control found that diabetic youths in single-parent families are generally in poorer health than those in two-parent families and have significantly higher levels of blood glucose when controlling for race, socioeconomic factors, and age of youth and of parent (Thompson, Auslander, & White, 2001). Social workers in community-based health care are in an excellent position to develop culturally responsive strategies to help at-risk families successfully adapt to the challenges of diabetic care for their teens and children. Disease management and educational interventions are effective in improving dietary and medication adherence, health outcomes, and quality of care, and in reducing the costs of care (e.g., Auslander, Haire-Joshu, Houston, Rhee, & Williams, 2002; *Diabetes Week,* 2004; Maljanian, Grey, Staff, & Cruz-Marino-Aponte, 2002; Philis-Tsimikas & Walker, 2001; Polonsky et al., 2003).

Pediatric Asthma

Pediatric asthma is the leading chronic illness in children affecting on average 6-8 percent, or 9.2 million children in the United States, and is increasing, particularly among minority children (American Lung Association, 2003). In some areas, specifically in inner city and urban centers, the rate of pediatric asthma is greater than 20 percent (Clark et al., 2004). The interaction of minority group status, socioeconomic factors, and medical factors is evident in the characteristics associated with asthma. Pediatric asthma is associated with

- the presence of allergies;
- a family history of asthma or allergies;
- low birth weight;
- being male;
- being black;
- living in a low-income environment.

In general mortality rates for asthma are highly correlated with living in poverty. Poor children and minority children with asthma are more likely to have limited access to health care, and less likely to receive high-quality and continuous medical care than nonpoor and non-Hispanic white children (Akinbami & Schoendorf, 2002; Tinkelman & Schwartz, 2004).

Asthma is a chronic, lifelong disease of the bronchial tubes (i.e., the airways of the lungs). For persons with asthma, these airways constrict, thus impairing the passage of air and, consequently, breathing. Pediatric asthma—asthma with onset in childhood—tends to be more difficult to control and effectively treat than asthma with first occurrence in adulthood.

Pediatric asthma affects the daily life of the affected children and their families because acute episodes, or asthma attacks, are life threatening. Families' responsibilities include monitoring the child for symptoms of attacks, incorporating strict medication regimens, and being vigilant of the child's environment at home, at play, and at school for respiratory irritants (i.e., allergens) that might trigger acute attacks.

Asthma is treated medically first by determining specific allergens, and then by providing medications that attempt to control allergic responses and bronchial constrictions, and preventing acute attacks. Disease management and educational interventions that include or focus on family members, particularly when implemented in the children's schools, have proven to be effective in stabilizing pediatric asthma and reducing negative psychosocial and medical outcomes (Clark et al., 2004; Tinkelman & Schwartz, 2004; Webber et al., 2003).

HIV/AIDS

As noted earlier in this chapter, statistics for HIV/AIDS are incidence numbers, rather than prevalence rates, due to the confidentiality regulations of the infection and disease syndrome. The incidence of HIV infection and of AIDS diagnoses across racial categories, as depicted in Table 2.1, is racially disproportionate. Even more dramatic is the disproportionate incidence by gender with racial groups (Centers for Disease Control, 2003a). As an illustration, though African-American women are about one-tenth of the total female population in the United States, they comprise more than one-half of all women diagnosed with AIDS and with an increasing incidence rate. AIDS is the third most common cause of the death of African-American women between the ages of twenty-five and forty-five years. Boyd-Franklin (2003) describes the situation poignantly—for African Americans, AIDS is a multigenerational disease; the vast majority of caregiving for infected family members and their affected or infected children is by family members.

HIV is the virus that attacks the immune system by infecting a specific white blood cell (i.e., CD4+), depressing the immune system and, thus, impairing the ability of the body to fight infection and diseases, and causing AIDS. White blood cells are an important part of the immune system that helps fight infections. Being infected with HIV (i.e., HIV+), however, does not mean that a person has AIDS. Rather, AIDS is the last and most severe stage of the HIV infection. As the virus attacks and destroys CD4+ white blood cells, the immune system becomes less able to fight infection and disease. A diagnosis of AIDS is based on the presence of one or both of the following: an opportunistic infection or certain malignancies, and/or levels of CD4+ cells below 200 cells per microliter. An opportunistic infection, such as pneumocystis pneumonia, or a cancer, such as Kaposi's sarcoma, is a disease that would not develop in a person with an intact immune system (Centers for Disease Control and Prevention, 2003a).

Because of advances in the pharmaceutical treatment of HIV, the time that persons may live with an HIV infection is extending. Some HIV+ persons may live for several years or even decades before developing, or may never actually develop, AIDS. HIV/AIDS is transformed from a once short-term fatal illness to a serious long-term chronic disease. Treatment for HIV infection includes highly complex medical and medication regimens and stringent efforts to prevent or reduce the extent of complications. Long-term medical care for a condition that is stigmatized has significant psychosocial issues for individuals and families. Practitioners' diligence in helping consumers to overcome barriers to receiving needed care and their expertise in counseling that facilitates consumers' coping with the challenges, and is empowering, are indispensable to assuring quality of life.

In brief, diabetes, pediatric asthma, and HIV/AIDS are major chronic illnesses with multiple psychosocial, lifestyle, and family ramifications that disproportionately affect culturally diverse populations.

These effects include increased psychosocial stress, compromised lifelong well-being, and lifelong economic challenges to pay for and/or gain access to needed care, resources, and services. Social workers in ambulatory health care practice are integral to overcoming these challenges and barriers.

One additional disease and two health risk factors, each affecting large numbers of consumers and linked to minority group membership, are worthy of discussion for social workers in community health care. These are obesity, hypertension, and at-risk pregnancy.

Obesity and hypertension are each linked to negative health outcomes, such as stroke, diabetes, and heart disease; at-risk pregnancy has negative health outcomes for both mother and child. These conditions are of particular note for social work in ambulatory health care because each of the three is associated with socioeconomic disadvantage and with psychosocial and behavioral characteristics. The following discussion provides a brief overview of the prevalence of and current research on these three conditions.

Obesity

Obesity has reached epidemic proportions in the United States. The prevalence of obesity is increasing in the total population, including teens, children, and adults across all statistical racial categories (Crespo & Arbesman, 2003). Prevalence rates increased from one-fifth (22.9 percent) in data covering 1988-1994 to nearly one-third (30.5 percent) for the data covering 1999-2000 (Flegal, Carroll, Ogden, & Johnson, 2002). Obesity is defined by the CDC (Centers of Disease Control), the National Institutes of Health, and the World Health Organization as having a very high amount of body fat in relation to body mass as indicated by a body mass index (BMI) of thirty or higher. The BMI is a measure of an adult's weight in relation to his or her height.

Varying data collection methods and categories of analysis make discussing prevalence rates for obesity by age, gender, and racial categories somewhat difficult. Therefore, the following discussion is based on best available estimates. The best estimates of prevalence rates among children and teens range from one-fifth (20.6 percent) for children two to five years of age, to nearly one-third (30.9 percent) for teens twelve to nineteen years of age (Crespo & Arbesman, 2003).

Minority women's rates of obesity are greater than for white women. Crespo and Arbesman (2003) suggest that the differences between culturally diverse and non-Hispanic white women evidences that obesity is related to socioeconomic class and education, with greater obesity associated with lower economic status and less education. Though the etiology of obesity is unclear at present, it is clear that rates of obesity are increasing in the United States, and that obesity is a risk factor for increased mortality, diagnoses of CVDs including hypertension and strokes, and diabetes.

Hypertension

Hypertension, or high blood pressure, in colloquial speech called "the silent killer," can affect anyone (American Heart Association, 2004). Hypertension can result in a cerebral-vascular accident (i.e., stroke), of which slightly over one-half are fatal. About one in every three adults in the United States has high blood pressure, occurring more often in men than women, and with greater rates in the southeastern United States than other regions. Rates of hypertension vary by race. For instance, among adult men, considerably more black (41.8 percent) people than whites (30.6 percent) and Mexican Americans (27.8 percent) are diagnosed with hypertension (American Heart Association, 2004).

The vast majority of hypertension diagnoses are of unknown etiology; most consumers diagnosed with hypertension have no symptoms whatsoever. However, even though many times high blood pressure does not have a known cause, it can be treated effectively with a combination of lifestyle changes and medications. A variety of differing medications treat the high blood pressure directly, or the underlying causes when known. Obesity, a physically inactive lifestyle, and high fat intake are associated with hypertension, Therefore, behavioral changes and lifestyle changes, including adhering to a low sodium diet, exercising, smoking cessation, losing weight, avoiding excessive alcohol intake, and stress management, can be effective interventions.

At-Risk Pregnancy

While the adolescent pregnancy rate in the United States decreased in the 1990s, the rate continues to be more similar to that of third world countries than other industrialized nations. Furthermore, the pregnancy rates for some minority adolescents in the United States actually increased during that same decade (Harris & Franklin, 2003). Research indicates that increased risk for a medically complicated pregnancy and delivery and increased risk of infant mortality are associated with mothers who are younger, poorer, less educated, single, and of a racial/ethnic minority (Berger, 2001; Centers for Disease Control, 2002a; Sharma, 1998). Medically complicated pregnancies are associated with high-risk, complicated delivery; poor birth outcomes; and maternal emotional and psychological well-being; and long-term developmental challenges for the child (Mason et al., 2001).

Unfortunately, though at-risk pregnancy programs and interventions are widely implemented, maternal and child health and social service systems are fragmented and replete with barriers to access to care (Bennett & Kotelchuck, 1997; Harris & Franklin, 2003). One of these barriers is the scarcity of culturally and linguistically responsive programs. Recommendations for better quality and access to maternal health care include involving community providers in planning, expanding maternal medical care to comprehensively include psychosocial services, and community-based health programs (Cunningham & Zayas, 2002). Community health social workers can achieve these objectives in program development and respond to research findings suggesting that participation in social support and educational prenatal and postnatal groups can lead to positive maternal psychosocial and health outcomes (Logsdon & Davis, 2003; Navaie-Waliser, Martin, Tessaro, Campbell, & Cross, 2000).

THE UNDERINSURED AND THE UNINSURED

Increases in the uninsured/underinsured population are racially disproportionate. Among the increases in the overall rate of uninsured Americans, African Americans and non-Hispanic whites had the most significant increases in 2002 (ABC News, 2002). According to 2002 data, over one-third (33.8 percent) of the Hispanic-American population, nearly one-fifth (19.3 percent) of black Americans, and one-fifth of Asian Americans (17.2 percent) were uninsured compared to 15.3 percent of non-Hispanic whites (U.S. Census Bureau, 2004).

Because many of the newly uninsured became so either as a result of losing their jobs—due to downsizing and/or layoffs—or to welfare reforms, the majority of the newly uninsured, and of the ongoing uninsured, are young adults, who do not qualify for any public assistance. Among the uninsured, the largest age group is between eighteen and twenty-four years of age (28.2 percent; Centers for Disease Control, 2002b), reflecting some consequences of welfare reform. Welfare-to-work reforms, though increasing the proportion of employment among the previously welfare dependent, most often result in employment that is low paying, less than full time, and/or without the availability of health insurance benefits. Thus, welfare reforms have increased in the number of Americans who are without health insurance (Weissman, Witzburg, Linov, & Campbell, 1999).

The number of underinsured health care consumers (i.e., those with insurance only for major medical with very large annual out-of-pocket expense requirements) is also on the rise. Being underinsured is related to consumers' income level, and the cost of the health insurance for both employers and consumers. Between 2002 and 2003, health insurance premiums increased nationally by nearly 14 percent (Kaiser Commission on Medicaid and the Uninsured, 2004). The cost of insurance may motivate potentially insured employees to reduce the extent of coverage they purchase and/or prompt employers to limit the insurance benefit offered. For those on limited or fixed incomes these factors, and therefore access to health care, are obviously exacerbated.

Research findings demonstrate the interaction of racial group and socioeconomic status in relation to being without health care coverage. For instance, Cornelius (2000) linked health insurance disparities of Hispanics in comparison with other racial groups to differences in income, the type of obtainable jobs, geographic mobility, ambivalence to seek health care due to immigration status, and overt employment discrimination. In addition, both public and private insurance and managed care companies may exclude some Hispanics. Concerning the latter, the Medicaid reform portion of the Balanced Budget Act of 1997 excluded coverage for certain classes of documented and undocumented immigrants.

The numbers of uninsured/underinsured in rural areas and in some regions of the United States are also disproportionate to the total population of these areas and regions. For instance, rural areas have 20 percent more of their residents without any health insurance and with only limited coverage compared with urban areas. Regionally the South (20.2 percent) and the West (8.8 percent) have greater proportions of the uninsured and underinsured in their populations than other regions of the country (Centers for Disease Control and Prevention, 2002b; National Rural Health Association, 2003).

Consequences of Being Uninsured or Underinsured

Those with health insurance coverage tend to believe that the uninsured are able to get care from hospitals and physicians, and that their care is either free or they are somehow able to pay out of pocket. However, research findings suggest that having no insurance is itself a barrier to accessing health care and that the costs of receiving health care are not easily paid by the uninsured (Van Loon, Borkin, & Steffen, 2002). That is, an estimated one-third to slightly more than one-half of the uninsured reported that they simply forego or cannot acquire care when needed. The uninsured use significantly fewer hospitalizations and physician visits than those with insurance coverage, a pattern that persists when all other demographic variables are controlled, and that is only slightly ameliorated as illnesses become increasingly severe (Hafner-Eaton, 1994; Van Loon, Borkin, & Steffen, 2002). In comparison with Americans with health care coverage, the uninsured and underinsured not only have restricted access to health care and may be less likely to get needed care, but also are in poorer health (Bertera, 2003; Donelan et al., 1996).

In examining how health care consumers perceive their choices concerning accessing care, Van Loon and colleagues (2002) reported racial differences in responses to the question, How much choice do you have about getting the health care you need? Nearly one-third of ethnic and racial minorities in the study responded that they had "little or no choice" compared to 16 percent of non-Hispanic white respondents. In addition, those without health insurance were less likely to seek physician visits even when all demographic variables were controlled—a finding that held whether the health condition was acute or chronic, or the uninsured person was healthy. While most uninsured in the study were employed, their employers did not offer insurance or employees could not afford the premiums. Anticipation of the cost of getting health care prevented over one-half from seeking needed care, even in instances of severe pain and injury, and over one-third reported going without needed prescriptions. When illness occurred, individuals utilized a comparative analysis to resolve whether or not to seek formal health care that followed these questions:

- How sick am I?
- Can I get by without health care for this illness?
- What home remedies can I use?
- Do I know anyone who has the medicine I need?

To sum up, this process of analysis involves comparisons of one's degree of illness and alternative sources of medication, and the cost of seeking formal medical care. Being uninsured or underinsured are barriers to receipt of health care that are not easily overcome, and compromise health. The increasing number of under- and uninsured—nearly one-fifth of the adults under sixty-five years of age without insurance, either public or private—face barriers and unpredictability in a system of health care that is at best arbitrary regarding gaining access to care.

HEALTH CONDITIONS AND PSYCHOSOCIAL FACTORS AND BEHAVIORS

Recent empirical knowledge has increased attention to the relationships of social and cultural characteristics, behavior, general health, and specific health conditions (Institute of Medicine, 2001). For example, Thompson and colleagues (2001) found significant relationships between the health status of diabetic youth and the structure of their families (Thompson, Auslander, & White, 2001). In addition, other findings suggest that effective diabetes management and physical outcomes are related to coping style, with coping styles varying by culture, gender, and race (DeCoster & Cummings, 2004; Willoughby,

Kee, & Demi, 2000). As a last example, CVD is related to both obesity and hypertension; obesity and hypertension are each related to dietary and physical activity patterns (Crespo & Arbesman, 2003). In brief, evidence suggests that psychosocial factors and behaviors are closely linked with disease and disease status.

SUMMARY

This chapter discussed the growing multiple and interactive trends in the health care consumer population including

- increasing longevity and diversity;
- consistent health disparities for minority consumer populations;
- increasing numbers of chronically ill consumers especially among diverse populations;
- increasing numbers of underinsured and uninsured health consumers;
- empirical evidence of relationships between psychosocial characteristics, behaviors, and health.

Changes among the health care consumer population require that social workers in community-based health care are knowledgeable and skilled in several areas of practice. One of the foremost needs is for culturally competent practice with individual consumers, and on behalf of groups or populations of consumers.

DISCUSSION QUESTIONS
AND ACTIVITIES FOR INDIVIDUALS
AND SMALL GROUPS

1. Given the disparities in health status, access to health care, and resources for health care discussed in this chapter, describe your vision for reconciling the social and economic justice issues for the growing population of consumers with limited coverage, access, and resources for health care. (*Hint:* Universal care might be an option, but is generally considered a "no go" in our society given the influence of special interests groups and our capitalist economy.)

2. What are the social and individual values attached to HIV/AIDS in your community? What are yours? How can the conflicts between these social and individual values and the needs of HIV-infected persons, AIDS consumers, and those affected by the virus and disease be addressed in your community? What groups and organizations might be helpfully influential in the resolution?
3. Engage in a discussion with people who have a chronic illness concerning the impact of that illness on their relationships, home life, sexual activity, and work; how they cope; and their experiences with health care systems and providers.

GLOSSARY

AIDS: Acquired immunodeficiency syndrome; caused by the human immunodeficiency virus and is the last stage of HIV infection; AIDS is diagnosed when an individual has one or both of the following: CD4+ cell count below 200 cells per microliter (μL) of blood and/or the presence of an opportunistic infection (such as pneumonia) or cancer due to an impaired immune system.

asthma: A chronic disease of the bronchial tubes (i.e., the airways of the lungs) characterized by tightening of these airways.

chronic illness: A serious, ongoing health condition that has a biological, anatomical, or physiologic basis and has lasted, or is expected to last, at least one year.

diabetes: A disorder of the body's ability to utilize glucose (i.e., sugar) in the blood.

epidemiology: The study of the frequency and distribution of diseases and disease patterns taking into account variations in geography, demographics, socioeconomic status, and genetics.

etiology: The cause or causes of a disease or abnormal condition as well as the branch of medical science dealing with the causes and origins of diseases.

HIV: Human immunodeficiency virus; the virus that attacks the human immune system by infecting and destroying a specific white blood cell (i.e., CD4+); CD4+ cells are part of the immune system that fights infections; HIV causes AIDS.

hypertension: High blood pressure; indicated when blood pressure frequently goes over 140/90 mm Hg (i.e., measured in millimeters [mm] of mercury [Hg]).

incidence: The number of newly diagnosed cases of a disease within a period of time (e.g., year, month, etc.).

morbidity: Any departure, subjective or objective, from a state of physical or psychological well-being; may be expressed as a proportion of persons per 100,000 persons with a particular diagnosis or condition.

mortality: The number of deaths in a given year per 100,000 persons in a defined population; the measure of the occurrence of death in a defined population during a specified interval of time.

prevalence: The proportion of a population having a disease, diagnosis, or medical condition over a specific period of time (e.g., year) expressed in a percentage.

renal: Pertaining to the kidney.

risk factor: An established direct cause of, or contributor to, the morbidity or mortality of a particular diagnosis or medical condition.

sequela(ae): An aftereffect of a disease, injury, procedure, or treatment.

underinsured: Having only major medical insurance, or having less than full health care insurance coverage.

uninsured: Having no health care insurance coverage.

Chapter 3

Cultural Competence in Ambulatory Health Care Practice

- *Why is understanding culture and cultural background important?*
- *What is culturally responsive practice in community-based health care?*
- *Are health disparities linked to cultural background?*
- *How can cultural background for practice be understood?*

INTRODUCTION

With the increasing diversity of the population, understanding the cultural background of clients and culturally competent health care practice gained a good deal of attention during the last two decades. While an in-depth discussion of cultural background is well beyond the scope of this text, understanding cultural background in relation to health, illness, and health care treatment and services is a prerequisite for culturally competent practice in ambulatory health care.

Understanding cultural background is necessary to effective engagement, assessment, and intervention with diverse health care consumers because culture may shape their experience of illness, and influence their interactions with Western, biomedically trained health providers and care. Research findings indicate that differing understandings, expectations, and beliefs about health, illness, and medical

Social Work Practice in Community-Based Health Care
© 2007 by The Haworth Press, Inc. All rights reserved.
doi:10.1300/5273_03

treatment between providers and health care consumers lead to frustration for all participants, complications in medications and diagnosis, and treatment avoidance and/or dropping out of care (Murguia, Zea, Reisen, & Peterson, 2000; Pachter, 1994; Pachter, Cloutier, & Bernstein, 1995).

The responses of the NASW on cultural competence in practice are indicative of its importance to the profession (National Association of Social Workers, 2001). In addition, the federal government established standards of cultural competence for health care and set cultural competence as a major national goal in the Healthy People 2010 plan (U.S. Department of Health and Human Services, Office of Minority Health, 2001; U.S. Department of Health and Human Services, 2002).

It is also important that community health practitioners realize that the dominant culture in the United States is a culture; it has values, norms, expected behaviors, and traditions (e.g., individualism, adherence to the importance of timeliness and efficiency, a future orientation), and that these are imbedded in Western health care systems, training, and practice.

Accordingly, this chapter explores culturally competent practice, health disparities, and cultural diversity, and it provides a framework for understanding consumers with culturally diverse backgrounds in the context of Western medical care; applications to practice in community health are interspersed as appropriate.

WHAT IS CULTURALLY COMPETENT PRACTICE?

What, then, is culturally responsive, or culturally competent, health care practice? The NASW describes cultural competence as practice that recognizes and affirms the value of diversity in culture, language, socioeconomic class, race, ethnicity, religion, and other factors. Culturally competent social workers have the capacity for cultural self-assessment and the consequences of the dynamics when cultures interact. The NASW (2001) includes the following as requisites for ethical culturally competent practice:

- specialized professional knowledge of the traditional values, family systems, and artistic expressions of major diverse groups and to integrate and transfer knowledge into standards, policies, and practices;

- skills, methods, and techniques that reflect the role of culture in the helping process and for empowerment, advocacy, and leadership on behalf of diverse clients;
- the attitude necessary to increase quality and better outcomes for diverse consumers.

The U.S. Department of Health and Human Services' National Standards on Culturally and Linguistically Appropriate Service (CLAS) reflects similar concepts specifically about health care (Thobaben, 2002; U.S. Department of Health and Human Services, 2001). The standards include ensuring that patients/consumers receive effective, understandable, and respectful care from all organizational staff members, and that care is provided in a manner compatible with their cultural health beliefs, practices, and preferred languages (Standard 1).

Culturally competent or culturally responsive practice is defined as a set of behaviors, attitudes, knowledge, skills, and policies that enables the work of agencies, organizations, programs, and professionals in cross-cultural provider–health care consumer interactions to be effective (Campinha-Bacote, 2002; Chin, 2000; Leininger, 1991; Panos & Panos, 2000). In brief, as described by Weaver (2005), cultural competence makes the work of the helping professions "more relevant to diverse populations" (p. 63).

Becoming culturally competent does not occur in an instant. It begins with practitioners understanding their own cultural background and, specifically for workers in health care, their own culturally related health beliefs, and the Western model of health care. Becoming culturally responsive assumes that the practitioner is willing to learn from health consumers and to understand the norms, social/family roles, values, and beliefs of diverse cultures, and is committed to engaging in cross-cultural experiences. The first step is understanding that there are a variety of worldviews, social structures, beliefs, and values among cultures and cultural groups (Campinha-Bacote, 2002; Congress, 2004).

The importance of knowing that all groups or populations are heterogeneous, rather than homogeneous, cannot be overemphasized; there is more within-group variation than between-group variation across and within all cultural backgrounds (Campinha-Bacote, 2002; Lum, Chang, & Ozawa, 1999). For example, each of two health care consumers might be Latino. However, one could be born in this country to Mexican-born parents, and the other arrived from Puerto Rico four months ago. Not only are these two clients likely to vary in terms of culturally related norms, traditions, social rules, and values, but they will also vary in culturally related health beliefs and the extent of assimilation to the Western biomedical model.

In summary, the cultural competence in health care centers on

- the practitioner's open and inquiring stance for learning from diverse consumers;
- a commitment to providing care within the context of the consumer's cultural background, health beliefs, and health practices.

Skills include the ability to collect information pertaining to consumers' cultural traditions, values, social/family roles, and health care beliefs; understanding of their current illness and its causality; and preferences for medical treatment (Campinha-Bacote, 2002).

WHAT ARE "CULTURE" AND "CULTURAL BACKGROUND"?

Several terms are used in the literature in any discussion of culture. In this text, the terms "culture" and "cultural background" are used interchangeably throughout. These concepts may be conceptually defined as the means of understanding one's world and life events—a lens that guides our thinking and ways of interacting with others. Culture is shared, learned, passed on from one generation to another by different groups of people and provides a reservoir of beliefs, social norms, roles and institutions, and values (Imes & Landry, 2002; Weaver, 2005). Culture is not static, but fluid, and changes with time, and in interactions with other cultural perspectives, particularly that of a dominant culture. That is, in the midst of a dominant culture, nondominant cultures are influenced by the dominant norms, values, social expectations and institutions, and language. Elements of cultural background, such as family structure, spiritual orientation, and social values, interact with each other to shape one's ways of understanding and of interacting in the world, expectations of one's own and others' behavior; provide coherence in making sense of life events; and influence consumers' experiences of health, illness, and interactions with health care providers.

Terms and Concepts for Understanding Cultural Background

A word of caution is warranted regarding categorical terms relating to diversity because many are used in the literature and professionally both inconsistently and interchangeably. It is generally accepted that official census data labels (e.g., African American, non-Hispanic whites, Hispanic) and others, such as Arab American or Southeast Asian, are socially constructed, too broad assuming that groups are homogeneous, and, as such, inadequate in and of themselves to the tasks of understanding cultural backgrounds and interpreting research findings (La Viest, 1994; Weaver, 2005). Furthermore, generalizations about cultural groups are not productive in establishing worker-consumer relationships or in understanding diverse consumer populations and communities (Congress, 2004). Accordingly, categorical labels such as those noted earlier are used when reporting findings of others who use those terms. In other discussions in this book, terms are used in respect to preferences of some groups, such as Latino, or Latina when referring specifically to Latino women, First Nations people, or black (Weaver, 2005). Last, in this discussion, the process of internalizing the values, norms, and so on of a culture—one's own or another—is interchangeably referred to as acculturation and assimilation.

First, however, any discussion of cultural background and cultural competence in practice with health care consumers should begin with health disparities.

HOW ARE HEALTH DISPARITIES LINKED TO CULTURAL BACKGROUND?

The concept "health disparities" refers to the gaps between majority and minority populations in health status, access to health care, and health care outcomes (Institute of Medicine, 2002). The term "health status" refers to the presence of a current illness. Health disparities exist for all minority populations across the lifespan. Research findings suggest that all minorities are more likely to receive lower quality health care and have higher mortality rates than non-Hispanic whites even when health coverage/insurance, income, age, and severity of health conditions are controlled (Institute of Medicine, 2002; Sudha & Multran, 2001; Thobaben, 2002).

Several causes for health disparities are suggested. In brief, disparities may be linked to cultural background, institutional intolerance, health consumers' lack of trust in health care providers, institutional bias, and/or stereotyping by providers and/or the interaction of socioeconomic status and culture (Congres, 2004; Gorin, 2001; Lums, Chang, & Ozawa, 1999; Thobaben, 2002). In regard to the latter, minority group health status is statistically related to greater likelihood of being poor and less educated than in the dominant culture's population. Substantiating this contention is the finding that economically poor health care consumers, who often lack health insurance, and are disproportionately of minority racial groups, have less access to health care and are in poorer health (Van Loon, Borkin, & Steffen, 2002).

A FRAMEWORK FOR UNDERSTANDING CULTURAL BACKGROUND

Because culture is fluid and there is more diversity within a particular population or group than between populations or groups, a conceptual framework for understanding culture is more useful than are listings or encyclopedic details of cultures (Weaver, 2005). To accomplish that objective the framework presented in this chapter incorporates elements that are common to human experience and that collectively comprise a cultural background and identity for each of us. Health care consumers of a specific cultural background may then be understood in light of a single or multiple elements.

As an illustration, the concept "family" organizes daily life on the individual, family, and social levels and, though varying in specifics, is an element of all cultures. Similarly, beliefs and understandings about what constitutes "health" and what constitutes "illness" as well as what causes illness, what are preferred treatments, and who are the preferred providers of treatments are present to some extent in all cultures, though heterogeneous within any one. Cultural groups have values, emphasize some values over others, and have social rules governing social interactions. In addition, spiritual orientation is part of human existence across cultures; sometimes a spiritual orientation may be reflected in the doctrine of a specific religion or prevalent in a particular cultural background or population.

Bearing in mind that the elements of cultural background are multiply interactive, and that heterogeneity within cultures and cultural groups is the norm, rather than the exception, the following sections discuss elements that are common in human experience across cultures and cultural backgrounds. The major elements of cultural backgrounds in this discussion are spiritual orientation; health beliefs; family; sexual orientation; acculturation; and social rules and values. These elements are depicted in Exhibit 3.1.

EXHIBIT 3.1. Elements of cultural background.

Spiritual Orientation

Control and Influence
Relationship

Health Beliefs

Causality of Illness
Concept of Health
Treatment and Care

Family

Structure
Authority
Roles

Sexual Orientation

Acculturation

Social Rules and Values

Spiritual Orientation

In this discussion, spiritual orientation is differentiated from religion and denomination, though several religions may have a similar spiritual orientation. The term "denomination" or "religion" refers to identification with a particular social institution (e.g., Presbyterian or Judaism) that has an organized set of beliefs, rituals, and behaviors that often includes officially sanctioned roles for leaders, activities, and doctrine. One's spiritual orientation furnishes a way of relating to other humans and the world in general, and making meaning of life. Spiritual orientation concerns one's worldview, and viewpoint in general about a transcendent control or influence in human life, an intrinsic human experience, conceptually defined as an internal, personal sense of connectedness to a higher or transcendent power(s) and others (Dosser, Smith, Markowski, & Cain, 2001; Van Hook, Hugen, & Aguilar, 2001).

In some instances, a spiritual orientation or a specific religious denomination may predominate in a particular culture. When a spiritual orientation, or a denomination for that matter, and a culture are colocated they are likely to have common characteristics. For example, those of the Hindu faith are predominately found in populations from India; thus, the Indian culture and Hinduism share social and familial characteristics (Hodge, 2004). In other instances, several cultural groups may share similarities in spiritual orientation (Dhooper, 2003; Murguia, Zea, Reisen, & Peterson, 2000; Weaver, 2003). As an illustration, some cultural groups such as Native American and Latino populations differ in many ways from each other and internally. However, the spiritual orientations of each stress harmony with all of life; the primacy and influence of an internal, personal path to and relationship with the universe; and a personal, internal relationship with spiritual ancestors and guides. In contrast, influence and control in human life may be fully in external and specific power(s) (e.g., god(s), fate, spirits, and God, Buddha, respectively).

What is important to understand about health care practice is that an individual's or a family's views on health and illness may relate to spiritual orientation and/or religious doctrine. As an example, in some spiritual orientations, illness is a punishment for sins, or victimization by an external force, or as part of a divine plan—in each case power resides in one or more external powers (e.g., Al-Krenawi & Graham, 2000b; Blackhall et al., 1999; Dhooper & Tran, 1998; McEvoy, 2003; Ow & Katz, 1999). In those circumstances, consumers may not see themselves as having influence or control over health or illness. Health care consumers with strong beliefs that externalities control illness and health may have conflicts with health care from Western biomedical providers, or may not see the worth of participating in their own health care plans and treatments.

Consumers who believe that power in human life is partially individual and partially in the hands of a higher, universal, or supernatural power may, on the one hand, seek help during times of illness from that higher power, while also participating actively in determining health care and care decision making (Van Hook, Hugen, & Aguilar, 2001). The challenge for practitioners is to understand and respect consumers' orientation and self-determination, while helping them participate in their medical care.

The reader is again cautioned to not overgeneralize particular spiritual orientations or religious affiliations with specific groups in the following discussion. Attribution of control to a transcendent being capable of solving human problems including illness is characteristic of the spiritual orientation of many groups. For example, the majority of black Americans are affiliated with conservative or fundamentalist Christian denominations, most notably Baptist and American Methodist Episcopalian denominations (McEvoy, 2003; Weaver, 2005). The spiritual orientation of fundamentalist denominations tends to affirm that the power to heal resides with God, healing occurs through prayer, and God can work through medical professionals (Van Hook, Hugen, & Aguilar, 2001). In addition, faith and church participation is central to the daily life of many African Americans; practitioners in ambulatory health need to incorporate that tendency in assessment and, when indicated, interventions (Billingsley, 1999; Boyd-Franklin, 2003).

First Nations people, members of some five hundred tribal affiliations, may vary in some details of their spiritual orientations, but hold certain precepts in common (Voss, Douville, Soldier, & Twiss, 1999; Weaver, 2003). In general, the spiritual orientation of Natives is centered on a harmonious integration and interactions of body-mind-spirit with all other life forms, including all of nature, the Creator, ancestral spirits, spirits of the natural world, and the connection and in relation to all other parts of creation. In general, Native Americans value the individual's spiritual life or path, while also placing great importance on the collective family, clan, and tribal spiritual experience. Spirituality is inseparable from physical, emotional, and mental health, and illness.

The spiritual orientation reflective of Judeo-Christian traditions typically involves a higher power, God, and in some instances includes other revered individuals (e.g., saints). Within this orientation are multitudes of specific religions and denominations. In general, the relationship of humans and God are specified in doctrine that may include a direct relationship of humans and God, or specify that the pathway to God is facilitated by another (e.g., priests). Latino populations are strongly influenced by a predominance of Roman Catholicism, with an emphasis on fatalism and a consequent belief that control is beyond the individual's grasp. Some specific Latino groups (e.g., Cubans, Haitians) also incorporate elements or blends of other spiritual orientations (e.g., African beliefs, or Voodoo and Santeria).

Prayer, meditation, and rituals and their implementation in daily life are, in general, specified religiously and denominationally and have implications for social work in community-based health care (Al-Krenawi & Graham, 2000b; Van Hook, Hugen, & Aguilar, 2001; Voss, Douville, Soldier, & Twiss, 1999). Many Christian blacks use prayer as a regular part of everyday life, rather than as part of official religious ceremonies alone, and as a coping strategy (Boyd-Franklin, 2003). Among the several doctrinal requirements for Muslims, prayer observance—a communal activity occurring in the context of multiple believers and at set times across the globe—is crucially important to their sense of overall physical, emotional, and mental well-being. Some Judeo-Christian denominations routinely provide meetings to pray (e.g., prayer circles) for congregation members who are ill. Native Americans tend to use activities, such as meditation and spiritual journeys, to integrate or heal the body, mind, and spirit.

Some recent research findings (Decoster & Cummings, 2004; McCullough, Hoyt, Larson, Koenig, & Thoreson, 2000; White, Townsend, & Stephens, 2000) suggest that prayer activities are related to positive health outcomes. These include a sense of wellness; positive responses to health care and treatment; and regaining health. Other findings are inconsistent suggesting that non-Hispanic whites utilize prayer more frequently than African Americans (Chadiha, Proctor, Morrow- Howell, Darkwa, & Dore, 1996). It is suggested that the inconsistency in research findings pertaining to the relationships of spiritual orientation, religion, religious practices, cultural background, racial groups, and health may result from cultural bias in research methodology and in the measurement of spirituality and religiosity (LaViest, 1994).

Health care practitioners are encouraged at a minimum to attend to the way that consumers describe their spiritual life. McEvoy (2003) suggests that, rather than generalizing associations of spiritual orientations or religions with certain cultural backgrounds, discussing the formal expressions of spiritual orientation, such as religious activities and affiliations, and how these beliefs are incorporated in a consumer's daily life provide the needed information and help establish an effective worker-consumer relationship. In summary, spiritual orientation gives meaning to life and can influence the experience of health and illness and consumers' views on their participation in medical care.

It is probable that practitioners may find the spiritual orientations of some cultural groups challenging when they differ from the worker's own. However, ethically responsible practice requires an open and inquiring stance regarding diverse spiritual orientations, and religious and denominational affiliations. Incorporation of this aspect of cultural background is essential to culturally competent practice in ambulatory health care programs with diverse consumers and in diverse communities.

Health Beliefs

Terms Related to Understanding Health Beliefs

Several terms appear in the literature in reference to health beliefs, including traditional medicine, ethnomedicine, ethnocultural medicine, and folk medicine, to refer to health care practices, products, and treatments of non-Western cultures/cultural backgrounds that are not currently accepted in mainstream Western medicine. These terms are used interchangeably throughout this chapter; culturally specific names for ethnocultural healers or physicians are used as appropriate. The dominant model of health care in the United States is known as the Western model of medicine, conventional medicine, allopathic, the biomedical model, as well as the "curative" model of medicine; these terms are also used interchangeably herein.

In the present discussion, health beliefs are defined as culturally related beliefs about the meanings and causes of illnesses, appropriate treatments, and the designation of appropriate health care providers and help-seeking health behaviors. Cultures vary in their beliefs about health, illness, and health care; the meaning of chronic illnesses; and how and when health care is sought. Therefore, understanding health beliefs is essential to effective social work practice in community-based health care given the poor health status, health disparities, and increasing number of cultural minorities in the health care consumer population (Brach & Fraser, 2000; Institute of Medicine, 2002; Lum, Chang & Ozawa, 1999; Sudha & Multran, 2001).

The Western Biomedical Model of Health and Illness

The Western biomedical model has a set of health care beliefs and standards of acceptable behavior, and it reflects the values and norms of the dominant culture in the United States (Imes & Landry, 2002). These values and norms are

- cause and effect thinking;
- positively valuing individual autonomy;
- positively valuing technology and efficiency.

Not surprisingly, the majority of health care practitioners, providers, and many, if not most, consumers in the United States believe in the biomedical model, and its values and norms. In order to understand how health consumers from non-Western cultural backgrounds may view and respond to the curative model of medicine, social workers in community-based health care need to understand the premises, values, and beliefs of the model.

The biomedical model rests on the "germ theory" of disease, where illnesses and diseases are understood as caused by contagion from bacteria, fungus, or virus, or by trauma, injury, aging, stress, or environmental agents or factors (Imes & Landry, 2002; Jackson, 1993). Diagnosis in this model requires identifying the causal agent of the dysfunction or illness; cause and effect links identify preferred treatments. Preferred treatments are interventions (e.g., antibiotics, chemotherapy, and surgery) directed at the cause (e.g., bacteria, injury). Healers are experts highly trained in the curative, Western model of medicine. Prevention of illness involves avoiding the causative agents, maintaining optimal physical activity and nutrition, and receiving Western health care.

Western medicine identifies some ethnocultural health care treatments as complementary, and as alternative to medical approaches, and defines these collectively as the practices, interventions, and treatments accepted by or included in the biomedical model. Ethnomedical interventions are often associated with one or more cultures or cultural backgrounds and may include massage; acupuncture; herbal remedies; techniques that enhance connection between physical body, mind, and the spirit; and dietary supplements. In some instances, traditional approaches have developed into health care systems, for example, homeopathic medicine and traditional Chinese medicine.

Because allopathic medicine is Eurocentric in its values and ideology, the role of individual autonomy, even decision-making authority, and participation in receiving health care is expected and valued (Aranda & Knight, 1997). In contrast, consumers of some non-Western cultural backgrounds are more likely to value collectivizing experiences, including receiving health care services and making health care decisions (e.g., Al-Krenawi & Graham, 2000a; Blackhall et al., 1999; Dhooper, 2003; Ow & Katz, 1999).

Some examples of the heterogeneity of health beliefs within cultures are useful at this point. Some specific Latino cultures, but not all, hold health beliefs that include the influence of supernatural powers, also known as magico-religious health beliefs, and disharmony on physical health to a greater extent than non-Hispanic whites (Murguia, Zea, Reisen, & Peterson, 2000, 2003). As a case in point, while a belief in voodoo as a cause and cure of illness is somewhat typical of those whose nativity is Haiti or Jamaica, it is not universally typical of all Hispanic groups (Murphy, 1993).

Patterns of the Use of Western and Ethnocultural Health Care

There are several patterns of the use of Western health care and folk medicine by consumers with non-Western cultural backgrounds. One pattern is the sole use of ethnocultural health care and traditional healers, and a second is the parallel use of folk medicine and indigenous healers, and Western medicine and practitioners. In addition, Western health care may be used sequentially when ethnocultural medicine and treatments fail. Last, culturally diverse consumers may choose traditional health practices for certain illnesses or health problems, and Western health care for others. As an illustration of the latter, Applewhite (1995) reports that older Mexican Americans choose *curanderismo* or choose Western medicine for treatment of illness by virtue of what care is accessible, what seems appropriate to the health problem they are having, and see no conflict in using both types of health care simultaneously. In another empirical study, Ma (1999) found that among Chinese Americans, a combination of traditional health remedies and Western health care is used. Americans of an Arab cultural background may use biomedical health care for physical illnesses and ethnocultural health care for emotional and mental problems (Weaver, 2005).

Interestingly, recent research suggests that alternative health care interventions are being used by more of the general population than might have been assumed (National Center for Complementary and Alternative Medicine, 2004). Alternative health care providers are also establishing themselves in both alternative and curative model health care centers. In the United States, in 2002, over one-third (36 percent) of adults reported the use of some type of complementary or alternative medicine, excluding megavitamin therapy and prayer, within the last twelve months, most often for chronic or recurrent pain control, colds, anxiety, and depression (National Institutes of Health, 2004; National Center for Complementary and Alternative Medicine, 2002). When prayer and meditation were included, nearly two-thirds (62.1 percent) reported use of alternative health interventions, with greater use reported by African-American (71.3 percent) adults.

Traditional, Ethnocultural Health Care

In traditional health care, health is most often defined in terms of the integration of the body, mind, and spirit, though the exact nature of each component, and how they interact, may vary across specific cultural backgrounds. Illness in ethnocultural perspectives is conceptualized as disequilibria, or the lack of harmony among body, mind, and spirit.

For example, Ow and Katz (1999) report that among Chinese Americans health is viewed as a state characterized by physical strength, sexual activity, virility, and fertility, rather than the Western view that health is the absence of illness. Traditional health beliefs—those associated with non-Western cultural backgrounds and groups—are conceptualized as naturalistic or as supernatural/magico-religious belief sets (Imes & Landry, 2002; Jackson, 1993). Some cultures' health beliefs fall into one or the other of these two categories, while others are a combination of the two. Each belief set will be discussed with examples of health beliefs and specific cultural backgrounds.

The Naturalistic Belief Set. In the naturalistic belief set, health is a balance or harmony of the body, mind, and spirit. In the naturalistic belief set, illness is caused by an imbalance of defined elements, such as excessive heat *(caliente)* or by excessive cold *(frio),* or imbalance in yin and yang, in the body (Imes & Landry, 2002; Jackson, 1993; Ma, 1999; Pachter, 1994; Pachter, Cloutier, & Bernstein, 1995). Excessive heat in the body may be caused by anger and result in a "hot" disease, such as hypertension. Excessive cold may result from eating too much cold food and cause "cold" illnesses such as of the gastrointestinal system. The goal of health care is to regain balance. Diagnosis involves identifying the hot or cold cause, and treating that imbalance, rather than the results or physical symptom(s) (e.g., hypertension) of the imbalance. The naturalistic health belief set is common in some Asian, Southeast Asian, Latino, and Native American groups.

Treatments of the naturalistic belief set include practices to restore balance such as herbal teas, tonics, massage, and acupuncture to reverse the imbalance of hot and cold, yin and yang, and so on (Ma, 1999). For example, Pachter and colleagues (1995) found that about one-fifth of Puerto Rican mothers used herbal preparations and syrups in treating asthma attacks (a "cold" illness) in their children.

"Cupping," applying suction to the skin, or "coining," rubbing the skin with a coin enough to cause bruising are also naturalistic belief set remedies (Jackson, 1993). In some Hispanic cultures, such as Mexican American, both these interventions are used (Galan, 2001). It is particularly relevant to social work in community-based health care to note that both cupping and coining may leave marks or bruises that can be misinterpreted by health care providers ignorant of their ethnocultural health treatment cause.

Supernatural/Magico-Religious Health Beliefs. The second health belief set in ethnomedicine is referred to as the supernatural, personalistic, or magico-religious belief set (Imes & Landry, 2002; Jackson, 1993). In this belief set, illness is caused by the active, purposeful intervention of another (e.g., person, god, ancestor, evil spirit). The ill person is essentially seen as a "victim" of the ancestor, evil spirit, and the like who imposes the illness by stealing, casting a spell over, or possessing the person's soul or spirit. Treatment involves identifying the supernatural being and rendering it harmless by lifting the spell, meditating, or inducing a trance. The healer, or the patient if he or she is believed to have the requisite power, can then overcome the supernatural influence. Symptoms of an illness are of only secondary concern. Prevention and good health are achieved by maintaining positive personal and spiritual relationships with both human ancestors and supernatural entities.

The supernatural health belief set may reflect spiritual orientation(s), and religious practices and beliefs. For instance, the cause of illness might be retribution for errant behavior by ancestors, gods, or God (Murguia, Zea, Reisen, & Peterson, 2000). Thus, by ensuring that one has not offended, or made anyone angry; avoiding the resentment of others; attending to culturally designated spiritual/religious rituals; and using protective spells one can assure maintaining good spiritual, mental, and physical health. For some who believe that illness is divine punishment and that healing is achieved only through faith, acceptance of and participation in Western biomedical care may be understood as showing a lack of faith.

Combining Naturalistic and Supernatural Health Beliefs

Some cultures combine natural and the supernatural belief sets in which illness is understood as having multiple causes, including an imbalance of yang and yin (i.e., female and male energy, respectively); a failure of harmony with the natural world; an obstruction of *chi* (i.e., life force); a curse by an offended spirit; or a punishment for bad behavior.

For several Latino cultures, folk medicine is referred to as *curanderismo,* also a combination of supernatural/personalistic and naturalistic health beliefs. *Curanderismo* involves a collection of beliefs and practices derived from ethnic and historical traditions that have as their goal the cure of psychological, spiritual, and physical problems (Applewhite, 1995; Murguia, Peterson, & Zea, 2003). *Curanderismo* often centers on a belief in God's divine will, while illness may be either natural or supernatural in origin. Healing is administered by those who have a divine gift, or *don,* and involves using herbs, candles, and prayer, recognized by a cultural community as specialized practitioners, known as *curanderos.* Other accepted healers include herbalists, bone/muscle therapists, and midwives. The use and extent of use of *curanderismo* varies in relation to availability, and acculturation to the dominant culture and the Western medical model of health care.

Native Americans' health beliefs can be described as a combination of naturalistic health beliefs, a spiritual orientation, and specific spiritual practices. Natives' spiritual orientation about human life includes the interaction of body, mind, and spirit; all of life is spiritually centered (Weaver, 2003). First Nations people generally expect that life naturally consists of what Western cultures might call negative experiences and problems (e.g., physical illness, spiritual crises, psychological or emotional problems). Accordingly, health care combines spiritual, emotional, psychological, and physical treatment; is holistic; and includes natural health belief set approaches. Health care practice includes the use of herbs, plants, and spiritual interventions, such as sweat lodges. Healers, who are called to be healers by the spirits of Native cosmology, and are highly revered, may be referred to as medicine men or women, and, in some tribes, as shamans. The role of healers is multifaceted including physical healing, psychological/emotional counseling, and spiritual guidance.

In brief, spiritual orientation is a component of cultural background, may be associated with particular cultural groups or backgrounds, and provides a way for humans to make meaning of life events, such as illness. The ways that persons participate actively, whether through religious and denominational organizations or privately, can be strengths and resources for coping with health problems.

Health Beliefs and Practice in Community-Based Health Care

Research findings suggest that a failure to take into account cultural health beliefs and care practices of consumers, such as alternative health care and treatments and their use, leads to miscommunication and misunderstandings, and may result in adverse medication interactions, diagnostic errors, and interrupted care (Brach & Fraser, 2000). Collaboration with traditional healers, and spiritual leaders as appropriate, is useful in ambulatory health care practice.

In summary, the singular construct of culturally related health beliefs is very informative but not sufficient by itself for culturally responsive practice in health care. In addition to understanding the spiritual orientation and health belief components of cultural background, practice must include knowledge of cultural background in relation to family structure, authority, and roles. These concepts are discussed in the following section of this chapter.

Family

Managed care's emphasis on consumer and family participation in care planning necessitates that practitioners are conceptually knowledgeable of the influence of cultural background on families in health care receipt. It is important to remember in this discussion that, as in all other components of cultural background, family structure, authority, and roles vary across, but more importantly within, cultures.

Structure

Family structure describes who is seen by the family as being a member. For purposes of this discussion, families are described as having a kinship/augmented, a clan/extended, or a nuclear structure.

The Kinship or Augmented Family Structure. A family with a kinship or augmented structure has members from multiple generations, who are biologically related, legally related, formally adopted, or informally adopted by a decision of the family, and who may also share a common ancestry or geographical nativity (Barnes, 2001). By way of a specific population example, black families are frequently described as having kinship/augmented family structures (Boyd-Franklin, 2003). Historically, many African-American families "took kids in"—informally adopted children who were sometimes biologically related, and sometimes not—in time of need and are more likely than whites to take in elders when the need arises (Boyd-Franklin, 2003). Members, though not biological or legally related to the family, are viewed as full family members and may be known, for instance, as "play sisters," "play mamas," or "play uncles" (Boyd-Franklin, 2003). Due to the importance that African-American families place on spirituality, members of their church are often included in their understanding of "who" is in the family (Porter, Gnong, & Armer, 2000; Williams & Dilworth-Anderson, 2002).

Augmented family structures may best describe families of attachment. Families of attachment are intentionally formed by their members, usually in combinations of partners, friends, and friends' friends, as epitomized in a recent successful sitcom. The concept references persons who are geographically and/or psychologically distanced from their families of origin, and is a preferred term among sexual minority populations (Schilder et al., 2001). In essence, families of attachment supply social support, as well as answer questions such as "Who am I?" and "Who is my family?" that any family structure does.

The Extended or Clan Family Structure. Cultures conceptualizing families as composed of persons who are biologically related and from multiple generations are characterized as having extended family structures. By way of illustration, First Nations people's families generally have extended family structures that include all those persons linked by matrilineal descent. All those related to the matriarch, or clan mother, are members of the family, or clan (Weaver, 2003; Weaver & White, 1997). One or more clans may comprise a specific tribe for some Native tribes, as well as for some Southeast Asian groups, such as the Hmong (Dhooper, 2003; Weaver, 2003). Overall, Asian families also tend to include persons across generations both vertically and horizontally within their extended family (Dhooper, 2003). An extended family structure, known as a *Hamula,* is culturally traditional for Arab families. A *Hamula* may constitute a tribal affiliation and is understood as those persons related biologically through patrilineal descent (Al-Krenawi & Graham, 2000a). Daily life for Arab families is dominated by interactions with both closely related and extended members of the *Hamula*.

The Nuclear Family Structure

The nuclear family structure may be perceived as typical of the dominant white culture in the United States; it may be more accurate to say that the nuclear structure in families is a stereotype, rather than a reality (Barnes, 2001). That is because culturally diverse families also have nuclear structures—particularly so with increasing mobility that may distance people from their larger family systems—while others may create a family of affiliation where they reside (Schilder et al., 2001). In its traditional form, a nuclear structured family generally includes two or at most three generations of biologically related persons (i.e., parents and child/children). In relation to practice in health care, nuclear families may not have the support systems in times of illness that is more characteristic of kinship and extended systems.

In community-based health practice, understanding whom the family considers as part of the family is necessary for effective engagement, assessment, and intervention. Applying the preceding discussion of family structure leads the practitioner to culturally salient approaches with health consumers and their families. To illustrate: in working with a consumer with a nuclear family structure, it would be appropriate to involve only parents and their children. Practice with a client from a culture characterized by a kinship/augmented structure might well require anticipating that family members not biologically related and/or from multiple generations would need to be engaged and involved in assessment and intervention. Specifically, inclusion of "church family" members might be crucial in working with African-American health care consumers and families. Similarly, practice with Native American consumers might best include the clan mother(s). Intervening with Arab-American and Asian-American health care consumers and families, consideration of the inclusion and acknowledgment of male authority members, possibly members from multiple generations, and incorporating tribal and/or community leaders in family interviews would be appropriate and helpful.

Authority and Roles in Families

The families of many non-Western cultures are hierarchical and have clear lines of authority and roles. For instance, in Arab, Asian, and Hispanic families decision-making authority tends to be male dominated, or patriarchal (Al-Krenawi & Graham, 2000a; Dhooper, 2003; Galan, 2001). In families from patriarchal cultural backgrounds, decision-making authority may move upward in the family system from one male to an older male, who is seen as having more authority. In considering consumers from cultural backgrounds that adhere to matriarchal leadership patterns, such as in several Native American tribes, authority in the family often rests with the oldest female clan leader, even when the official chief of the tribe is male (Weaver & White, 1997; Weaver, 2003).

Familism is associated with authority in families. Familism is conceptually defined as the strong identification, attachment, solidarity, and loyalty to the family, and reciprocal supportive relationships, with deference to the collective force of the family in decision making (Luna et al., 1996). The salience of familism varies across cultures, but is considerably more evident in non-Western cultures. Generally, familism is strong and collective responsibility for the well-being of family members is valued in Southeast Asian and Latino cultural backgrounds. Because African-American families view authority as collectively held in the family, and include church leaders or ministers as consultants in decision making about family members, the value placed on the individual autonomy of the patient may not be as primary a value as held in Western medicine. Families from Middle Eastern cultures may evidence strong both familial and tribal loyalties, and tribalism. Health care consumers of various cultural backgrounds that stress familism and health care providers from the Western curative model of medicine may have dissonant views about how health care decision making should occur.

In relation to the concepts of family structure, roles, and authority, it should be apparent that the belief that individual patient autonomy in health care decision making is primary, as held in both Western medicine and the dominant Western culture, is not necessarily reflective of all cultural backgrounds. By way of one illustration, research findings suggest that Mexican Americans and Japanese Americans believe that patients should not be told they are terminally ill, whereas both non-Hispanic whites and African Americans generally believe they should (Blackhall et al., 1999).

Gender roles are related to authority in families, as well. Gender roles are inclined to be clearer and fixed in non-Western, than in Eurocentric and dominant Western cultures. As an illustration of gender roles, Hispanic and Arab cultures have clear and overt gender expectations (Al-Krenawi & Graham, 2000a). Men are responsible for the family and hold status as the heads of families and in the community. Women are expected to focus their energies fully inside and may not be allowed to participate in activities outside the home. Conversely, women in the Native American culture are revered as and expected to be community and tribal leaders (Weaver & White, 1997). Gender roles in the dominant Western culture are generally more fluid and shift with more ease in response to external influences such as economics and the need to work outside the home.

Incorporating an understanding of the consumer's family structure, identifying who holds decision-making authority in the family, and gender roles will enhance the likelihood of effective engagement, assessment, planning, and intervention. Without this knowledge, workers may falsely assume that consumers' family structure and authority patterns are the same as their own, or tend to overgeneralize. Doing so can lead to an over- or underassessment of family strengths, stresses, social support resources and needs, and the readiness to comply with recommended interventions (Campinha-Bacote, 2002).

In summary, social work practice in health care necessitates consideration of a consumer's culturally related family structure, authority, and gender roles in assessment and planning interventions.

Sexual Orientation

Sexual orientation may well be at least as emotionally and politically charged as any other single aspect of cultural background and identity. Social, family, and individual attitudes about sexual orientation are influenced by spiritual orientation, specifically religion, family, and gender roles separately and in combination. It is beyond the scope of this text and chapter to explore the knowledge base about sexual orientation overall. Rather, the purpose is to discuss sexual orientation in relation to specific issues in health and illness and health care delivery for social work in ambulatory health care practice.

Terms Relating to Sexual Orientation

As in all areas of cultural backgrounds, terms related to sexual orientation change over time and are socially constructed. At present, sexual orientation is generally defined in terms of sexuality—sexual activity with one or both sexes. However, in some discussions the conceptual definition of sexual orientation includes an affectional orientation, thus broadening the definition. Sexual orientation includes heterosexuality (i.e., attraction to and sexual activity with persons of the sex other than your own), bisexuality (i.e., attraction to and sexual activity with persons of either or both sexes), homosexuality (i.e., attraction to and sexual activity with persons of your own sex), and transgendered (i.e., being born physically of one sex while psychoemotionally being of another). These various orientations are represented across and within cultures and cultural backgrounds, though they may be publicly lived more so in some than others.

Religion and denominational doctrine interact with gender expectations in views about sexual orientation across and within cultural backgrounds. For instance, Judeo-Christian religions tend to honor the primacy of a heterosexual sexual orientation, with some denominations more acceptant of other sexual orientations. However, some religions are overtly negative about any orientation other than heterosexuality. As an illustration, for African Americans who are widely associated with fundamentalist Protestant churches, the church's message may well be "compulsory heterosexuality" (Weaver, 2005, p. 117). As a result, blacks, including those of Caribbean nativity, of several Christian faiths tend to express homophobic attitudes. Green (1999) suggests that among African Americans cultural identity is a combination of race, gender identity, and sexual orientation. Green suggests further that, because of this combination, African-American lesbians and bisexuals experience multiple layers of oppression and stigma. Among Middle Eastern cultures, sexuality and gender is often determined by Islamic doctrine with rigid mandates and social approbations for any variation. First Nations people's viewpoints about sexual orientation reflect their belief that sexuality in all its forms is natural and sacred, and all sexual orientations are accepted (Weaver, 2005).

Being gay, lesbian, bisexual, or transgendered continues to be a politically and socially powerful component of cultural background, and unfortunately often an issue of social stigma. In terms of health care, most professionals, health care organizations, and systems reflect the heterosexist bias of the larger society, which has implications for health care consumers who are members of sexual orientation minorities, and practitioners. In addition, sexual orientation is rarely covered in allopathic medical education.

Research on the psychosocial and health care concerns of sexual minorities receives comparatively little attention. However, some empirical findings are available. For example, findings imply that, as with other cultural minorities, consumers who are gay, lesbian, bisexual, or transgendered frequently experience negative attitudes and prejudice from health care providers (Schilder et al., 2001). Specifically, findings of Schilder et al. include reports that some providers project their own heterosexual concepts, and prejudices about sexuality, on sexual minority consumers. Behaviors like those can diminish the willingness of clients to participate in their own health care and to disclose needed information to professionals. Health care organizations also reflect dominant social attitudes. Health systems often fail to include members of the families of attachment of gay, lesbian, bisexual, and transgendered persons in care and consent processes, seeking instead members of the consumers' family of origin.

Social workers in ambulatory health care are well placed to help colleagues without the necessary education understand the psychosocial and health issues related to sexual orientation. Education of interdisciplinary colleagues and advocacy on behalf of consumers demonstrate valuable expertise and professional ethics.

Acculturation

The increasing pace of immigration during the last two decades has resulted in an increasing proportion of health care consumers who are comparatively recent immigrants or have family members who are. Therefore, health practitioners need to understand the experience of acculturating to the dominant culture of the United States and the influences that bear on that process, because these can impact health and receipt of health care.

Acculturation is the process of internalizing a culture's beliefs, values, norms, expectations for behavior, and language, generally in reference to a culture other than one's own (Galan, 2001; Panos & Panos, 2000). Three aspects of acculturation are described in the literature: assimilated, bicultural, and traditional. Persons who are described as fully assimilated have incorporated the dominant culture's ways and values and seek to have all their social, psychological, political, and economic needs met in the dominant society. Those who adhere to their own culture's ways, norms, values, and language, while living within another culture, are described as cultural. Persons who maintain the norms, values, and traditions of their own culture while also internalizing those of another, usually a dominant culture, are described as being bicultural (Barrios & Egan, 2002; Weaver, 2005). Biculturalism, it should be noted, is not a term connoting a deficiency. Rather, being skilled in two or more cultures is valuable in an increasingly diverse society.

Another category of acculturation—liminalization—is also discussed in the literature (Panos & Panos, 2000). Liminalization is the experience of not being linked to one's own culture while also not linked to the culture of the dominant society either. Liminalization is akin to cultural disenfranchisement. Lum and colleagues (1999) report that both physical and mental illness are associated with cultural liminalization. As an illustration, because First Nations people often live away from Native communities or off the reservation, disjoined from family, clan, and tribal supports, it is suggested that liminalization may be a common experience for some Natives (Walters, 1999). Others suggest that Native Americans become skilled in biculturalism for economic reasons, and utilize their cultural and spiritual heritage, even if only privately, as strengths and coping mechanisms (Barrios & Egan, 2002; Weaver, 2005).

Understanding that acculturation and the formation of a cultural identity do not follow a uniform or linear path, it is clear that the length of time an individual resides in a dominant society, though relevant, does not indicate the extent of acculturation to the dominant culture (Panos & Panos, 2000). Persons may assimilate some of the majority culture's ways while maintaining their traditional culture's norms and values in other areas of their lives. One example will be illustrative. The Western majority culture's emphasis on individualism may be assimilated within the context of work, while collective-familial decision making, traditional health care methods, or language are maintained and used in the home. Murguia and colleagues (2000) report research findings suggesting that a greater maintenance of ethnocultural identification is related to lower utilization of Western biomedical health care and less compliance with health treatment recommendations of Western curative medical providers (Murguia, Zea, Reisen, & Peterson, 2000).

Immigration and Acculturation

Acculturation may be influenced by experiences before and during immigration and is related to acculturation stress (e.g., Congress, 2004; Dhooper & Tran, 1998; Galan, 2001; Panos & Panos, 2000). Acculturation stress is the degree to which energy must be expended to adapt to the immigration experience itself and to the new culture. Immigration stress is a function of the impact of crisis events surrounding the reason for and the process of immigration, the person's age at the time of immigration, and the nature of the individual's or family's interface with the dominant society in the process. That is, acculturation may be less stressful for those immigrating at younger ages, for those whose immigration was purely voluntary and not as asylum seeking, and for those who have no conflicts with the government or society of the dominant culture concerning their immigration process. Having a cultural network or community to embrace, where communicating in one's native language and celebrating familiar traditions and holidays is easy, can ameliorate some of the stress of the immigration and the acculturation experience (Kemper & Barnes, 2003).

Adjusting to the dominant culture in the United States is, nonetheless, inherently stressful. Arab immigrants, for example, are known to experience divided cultural loyalties, and to adapt biculturally, rather than to assimilate, to a greater extent than other immigrant groups (Al-Krenawi & Graham, 2000a). The biculturalism of Arab Americans of their own and the dominant culture may be affected by longer residence in the Western society, younger age at immigration, not recently visiting the native country, the condition(s) prompting immigration, the extent of local culturally responsive social support, and the degree of religious affiliation (Al-Krenawi & Graham, 2000a). In addition, Arab Americans may socially isolate and adhere to traditional cultural beliefs, values, and norms in response to media attention to their culture (Nobles & Sciarra, 2000).

In general, younger members of culturally diverse and immigrating families, because they attend public schools of the dominant society and thus are exposed to dominant cultural influences, may achieve biculturalism more quickly or readily than older family members. Galan (2001) discusses the disruption potential for Mexican- and Cuban-American families, and the burdening of their children and teens when social workers and other professionals depend on them to act as interpreters or to take on case management roles for the family. Such an approach is not by definition problematic but, if challenging family unity, structure, authority, or roles, may precipitate into family crises. Last, consumers who are recent immigrants may be reluctant to seek health care, or engage with practitioners, when legal status and/or stigma is associated with illness (Chillag et al., 2002).

In summary, in community-based health care social work with consumers who are immigrants to the United States, practitioners need attend to acculturation. Connections to culturally salient social support mechanisms, such as groups and communities, may help ameliorate the stress of illness and of interfacing with health care providers of the Western model of medicine. Incorporating the cultural resources and networks currently in use by the client and his or her family early in the information gathering process, appropriately determining whether and then, if appropriate, how to achieve connections to those cultural support mechanisms in care planning is important.

Social Rules and Values

The social rules and values of one's cultural background provide guidelines for human interactions and a sense of security during challenging events or crises. In the context of community-based health care, culturally diverse consumers are likely to draw upon the social values and rules of their traditional cultural background during illness, physically incapacitating events, and receiving biomedical health care because these values and rules assist in coping. The dominant U.S. culture values competition, meeting one's own needs, financial gain, personal ownership, the rights of the individual, and a future orientation both attitudinally and behaviorally. Not surprisingly, two of these values—the rights of the individual and a future orientation—are imbedded in the philosophy and expectations of what is "normal" consumer behavior in the curative medical model (Panos & Panos, 2000; Patcher, 1994).

One issue for practitioners of the dominant Eurocentric culture is understanding the potential conflict between individualism and the collectivism held in many non-Western cultures. As noted previously, Western health care can be described as a cultural group in that it has norms of behaviors, social roles, and values. One indicator of Western medicine as a cultural group is the primacy placed on individualism and the individual in health care. Accordingly, Western providers tend to ascribe to autonomy in health care decisions and planning, and responsibility for illness and health to the individual consumer. Health care providers adhering to individualism expect consumers to participate in health care planning, and to comply with medical regimens. Western health care providers may see this latter set of behaviors as normal, whereas pathologizing consumers hold that collective and familial decision making is normal (Panos & Panos, 2000; Zayas & Dyche, 1992). These discrepant expectations and values may promote multicultural consumers' distrust of Western health care providers, disrupt continuity of care, or prompt consumers to drop out of care.

Several cultures tend to have strong social rules concerning behavior that differ from and are generally more stringently adhered to than social rules in the dominant Western culture. For example, Chinese Americans' rules of social behavior emphasize saving face, maintaining group harmony and mutual protection—especially the family group—and adhering to hierarchical roles and respect for authority figures, such as physicians and health care providers. Social rules such as these are antithetical to Western medicine's expectations that consumers are assertive and proactive.

Social rules that predicate interactions on a hierarchical status also have implications for practice in community health care. Consumers with these social rules may demonstrate respect by politely deferring to physicians and by seeming to agree about diagnoses and planned care, whether or not they actually do agree or understand (Ow & Katz, 1999). They may be hesitant to ask questions, voice worries, or reservations. Consumer hesitancies such as these can interfere with establishing the trust necessary for effective provider-consumer relationship building. And, unfortunately, some research findings suggest that some culturally diverse consumers do not trust Western health care or physicians and, thus, may avoid an open discussion of their health concerns or simply not return for further care (Ma, 1999).

Understandably, consumers of cultural backgrounds with a history of being oppressed may be distrusting of relationships with health care providers and professionals of the dominant culture. As a case in point, black American clients may seem reserved, even appear aloof, when first meeting with health care professionals of the dominant culture, such as social workers. Formality may be an important social rule for consumers; respect is demonstrated by expecting to be addressed with formal titles (e.g., Mrs., Mr., Miss) (Boyd-Franklin, 2003). Caution in relating to the worker may reveal itself by checking out the worker's integrity and trustworthiness for some period of time or through a number of sessions. As often as not, however, once an African-American family fully engages, their relationship with the social worker is often one of high personal regard and longevity (Boyd-Franklin, 2003).

Social rules about nonverbal behavior are also culturally bound. For instance, crossing one's leg and letting one's foot point at another person is insulting in some Southeast Asian and Middle Eastern cultures (Weaver, 2005). American Natives' norms of nonverbal behavior such as avoiding eye contact and being silent can be perceived by Western practitioners as indicating psychological or self-esteem problems. Behaviors that show stoicism are highly valued in several Asian cultures. As a result, Asian Americans may be reluctant to acknowledge discomfort and pain even to their medical providers; physical pain may be seen, not as an aberrational health condition requiring intervention, as is true in Western medicine, but as a normal part of human life (Dhooper & Tran, 1998). For example, research findings imply that Chinese and Filipino Americans endure and accept higher levels of pain than non-Hispanic whites (Ow & Katz, 1999).

Differences in social rules and values held by allopathic practitioners and consumers from other cultural backgrounds can interfere with effective provider-client relationships. Western health providers may be unaware of culturally related behaviors; these may go unrecognized or misinterpreted by providers, undermining effective care provision.

Differences in the meaning of, and the importance placed on, "time" is a case in point. The dominant U.S. culture and the Western medical establishment adhere to the value of "clock time." Providing health care services is time bound; providers value punctuality and expect health care consumers to as well. Other cultures have differing concepts of time. Some Latino and Middle Eastern cultural groups tend to view time as less determined by the clock, and more to the social rhythm of day. Arab-American health care consumers are likely to view time as fluid, and expect that both the beginning of a session with a social worker and its conclusion are dependent on the collective agreement of those in the session. For Native Americans, time is generally seen as an endless continuum—a circle—that has no beginning, middle, or end. A family or community member's needs easily take precedence over arriving at a medical appointment on time. For consumers of various cultural backgrounds being "on time" is not a value that has priority in organizing behavior.

In addition, the Western culture and medicine tends to be future oriented, whereas some cultural groups are present oriented (Weaver, 2005). Thus, addressing current concerns is very important in engaging clients and families, though the practitioner may tend to think of interventions for longer term change. Understanding how the client or client's family views "time" is obviously salient to effectively engaging health care clients. Mainstream practitioners who do not understand the relevance of differing views of time and its importance in working with culturally diverse clients may negatively evaluate consumers on the basis of their punctuality to appointments, or miss the need to discuss the timing of medication regimens and treatments that may be longer term, such as behavioral changes in lifestyle, in culturally germane ways.

Values concerning elders and the process of aging itself also vary across cultural backgrounds. The Western dominant culture tends to see aging as a time of comfort and relaxation, with increasing frailty.

For instance, among Chinese or Japanese cultures, older adults are seen as becoming increasingly venerable as they age. Their wisdom is highly respected and elders are seen as guides for the family and the community. Some cultures specify social values and behaviors concerning elders and the role of younger family members regarding them. One example is *hyodo,* or filial piety, a social value strongly held in the Korean culture that obligates the family to do whatever is necessary to delay the death of elders (Blackhall et al., 1999). The implications for health care practitioners working with severely or terminally ill consumers and their families holding the value of *hyodo* are obvious.

In summary, health care consumers and families who hold the dominant culture's value of individual autonomy, meeting one's own needs, punctuality, and a future orientation may have less difficulty adapting to the norms and values of biomedicine than those whose cultural values are centered on sharing, family, and a fluid orientation to time.

SUMMARY

The cultural backgrounds of health care consumers are clearly relevant to practice in community-based health care settings. In summary, the foregoing sections of this chapter discuss dimensions of culture in relationship to health, illness, and health care and ethno- and Western medicine and suggest several areas needing attention by practitioners. These areas include

- spiritual orientation, religious affiliations, activities, and practices including the role of prayer/meditation;
- the definition of who is in the family and who makes care decisions;
- health beliefs, and possibly including ethnocultural health practitioners and religious leaders in interviews;
- the possible need for a language interpreter;
- acculturation and immigration issues;
- social rules and values.

In conclusion, these dimensions of cultural background are each vital for culturally competent practice in ambulatory health care.

DISCUSSION QUESTIONS AND ACTIVITIES
FOR INDIVIDUALS AND SMALL GROUPS

1. Use the elements of cultural background and the culturally related assessment topics and questions in Appendix C to describe each of the elements in your own cultural background.
2. Reflect on your self-assessment and present strengths and challenges facing social work practice with consumers with culturally diverse backgrounds. Are any elements particular strengths or challenges? Do these relate to specific backgrounds?

GLOSSARY

acculturation: The process of internalizing a culture's beliefs, values, norms, expectations for behavior, and language; also referred to as assimilation.

allopathic medicine/biomedicine/conventional medicine/curative medical model/biomedical model: Terms that are used to describe the Western model of medicine.

alternative medicine: Health care, treatments, practices, and products not currently accepted by the allopathic model of medicine.

bicultural: Maintaining the norms, values, and traditions of one's culture while also assimilating those of another, usually dominant culture.

complementary medicine: The combined use of the biomedical model and alternative health care.

curanderismo: Part of the magico-personalistic health belief set; collection of beliefs and practices derived from ethnic and historical traditions that have as their goal the cure of psychological, spiritual, and physical problems; generally associated with Latino cultures.

ethnocultural medicine/folk medicine/traditional medicine/ethnomedicine: Health care practices, products, and treatments of non-Western cultures/cultural backgrounds.

extended family: A family structure concept describing a family composed of persons who are biologically related and from multiple generations.

familism: The strong identification, attachment, and loyalty to the family, and reciprocity and solidarity among family members with deference to the collective force of the family in decision making.

health disparities: The gaps between majority and minority populations in health status, access to health care, and health care outcomes.

kinship/augmented family: A family structure concept describing a family with members from multiple generations, who are biologically related, legally related, formally adopted, or informally adopted by a decision of the family, and who may also share a common ancestry or geographical nativity.

liminalization: The experience of not being linked to one's own culture while also not linked to the culture of the dominant society.

morbidity rate: The proportion per 100,000 persons with a particular diagnosis or condition.

mortality rate: The number of deaths in a given year per 100,000 persons in a defined population.

nuclear family: A family structure concept describing a family with two or at most three generations of biologically related persons (i.e., parent[s] and child/children).

Santeria: A supernatural/personalistic health belief set associated with Caribbean cultures that includes practices to restore spiritual/physical/emotional well-being.

Western medicine: The dominant medical model; also referred to as allopathic medicine, biomedicine, conventional medicine, curative medical model, and the biomedical model.

Chapter 4

Social Work in Community-Based Health Care

- *What is social work in community-based health care?*
- *What is the history of social work in health and community care?*
- *In what settings does social work in ambulatory health care occur?*
- *What advances in communication technology are used in ambulatory health care?*

INTRODUCTION

As discussed in the previous chapters, the paradigm shift in health care moved care into the community, refocused care from acute to chronic illnesses, and transferred the authority for care delivery to managed care systems. Briefly, health care now focuses primarily on providing efficacious, short-term interventions in the community across a continuum of care for consumers with frequently predictable, largely chronic health conditions, and/or for defined consumer populations or conditions.

This chapter discusses social work in community-based health care in light of these transitions and ramifications for health care social work practitioners and consumers. Ambulatory health care practice affords both challenges and opportunities for practitioners and

Social Work Practice in Community-Based Health Care
© 2007 by The Haworth Press, Inc. All rights reserved.
doi:10.1300/5273_04

for consumers. Accordingly, the chapter explores social work practice in community health care in terms of emerging practice settings and social work roles, knowledge, and skills. Ethical considerations are incorporated as appropriate. But first, a discussion of some of the challenges and the opportunities for social work resulting from an unintended consequence of the paradigmatic shift in health care is warranted.

In response to the paradigm shift, there were widespread attempts by health care organizations to meet the cost containment criteria, while maintaining existent and capturing new market share. The unintended corollary of these efforts is fragmentation of health care delivery systems (Dziegielewski & Holliman, 2001). As a result, in order to receive care, health care consumers must traverse complex, but often disjointed, service delivery systems, moving sequentially from one health care organization or setting or provider to another. That is, a consumer receiving health care in one setting is, albeit benignly, "referred on" to other health care and social services. Unfortunately, those referred-to agencies often continue the referral pathway instead of, or in addition to, providing their services. Thus, intake, assessment, and referral are disconnected or redundant events with little or no recursive feedback. Figure 4.1 depicts such a pathway for one health care consumer.

Figure 4.1 suggests the interorganizational problems and the challenges to social work in ambulatory health care settings. Because health care systems are fragmented, and managed care emphasizes interdisciplinary coordinated care, practitioners must ensure a continuum of care with integrated health care. It is important at this point to clarify two descriptive terms frequently used in the literature. The term "interdisciplinary" is conceptually defined as the joint integrated efforts of all providers in care planning and delivery. In contrast, multidisciplinary care is developed and implemented by providers parallel to each other without integration. Multidisciplinary practice can be visualized as silos, or tall chimneys—each situated on a common base (the consumer) but with no interconnections or reciprocity. Professional turf conflicts, the need to maintain a market share, and/or revenue streams may foster the latter, while also promoting duplication of and gaps in services. The upshot for consumers is that acquiring needed care can be daunting, complex, and frustrat-

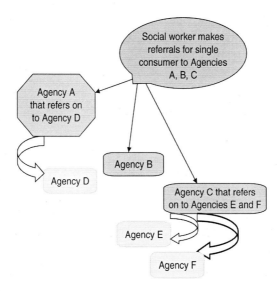

FIGURE 4.1. A fragmented consumer pathway.

ing. Essentially clients have to be their own coordinators in order to transit the pathway depicted in Figure 4.1. Social workers in ambulatory health care are uniquely prepared to facilitate that pathway for individual consumers and families, and to develop integrated programs and systems.

WHAT IS SOCIAL WORK IN COMMUNITY-BASED HEALTH CARE?

Social work in ambulatory health care is a practice that occurs outside of hospitals; connects people in a community with health care providers, resources, and services; and involves a spectrum of services from direct practice to program development, particularly for vulnerable, at-risk populations. Poole and Van Hook (1997) suggested that the revolution in health care would necessitate discovering and developing ways to replace "fragmented health care systems with coordinated networks of care" (p. 2) to address the needs of at-risk populations in practice that spans organizational boundaries and to "coordinate health services in accessible community sites" (p. 3).

In a similar vein, Rosenberg and Holden (1997) proposed that health care practice in the twenty-first century would combine indirect and direct practice roles in linking health care organizations and developing programs for at-risk populations, including prevention and health promotion. Corwin (2002) describes community-based health care as "ambulatory care" (p. 193), clearly differentiating community health care from both inpatient/institutional or hospital care and care for the homebound, such as hospice and home health.

Social work in ambulatory health care may be direct practice or practice on behalf of consumer populations. Direct practice activities center on a consumer's present health condition and address the psychosocial components of a health diagnosis, an exacerbation of an illness, and/or challenges arising from a chronic illness (Corwin, 2002; Dziegielewski & Holliman, 2001). On behalf of consumers, social workers engage in programmatic activities in the community among health organization providers, community groups, and stakeholder organizations to resolve fragmented health care systems and unmet population needs. In sum, community health care practice involves social workers in multiple roles, and in both direct and indirect practice activities.

Social work practice in ambulatory health care occurs in a variety of settings. Settings may have simple or complex organizational structures, and be nonprofit, public, or proprietary. Settings include, for example, individual and group physician practices, clinics, primary care, university-community and multicommunity agency partnerships, corporate, and FBOs. Clinics may be a component of public health departments, part of large hospitals or health care systems, or freestanding enterprises. Partnerships between universities and community entities and between multiple community organizations are responses to integrate fragmented health care delivery systems (Mosley, 1998; Poole & Van Hook, 1997). Funding sources for ambulatory health care settings, in singular and combined forms, include government grants and contracts, consumer generated revenue, community and congregational sponsorship, and third party payer coverage.

New opportunities for social work practice and leadership for general and specific consumer populations, in innovative programs targeting emerging consumer populations and to ameliorate the inequities and fragmentation of health care delivery systems, are growing (e.g., Galambos, 2003; Lesser, 2000). By way of just one illustration, research findings correlate social, physical, and dental health needs in populations that have little or no social, health, or dental care resources (Waldrop, Fabiano, Davis, Goldberg, & Nochajski, 2004). Social workers and dentists are collaborating in response to the unmet needs of this population in an urban school dental clinic. Social workers are training dental residents about child abuse/neglect, domestic violence, and the biopsychosocial perspective of health care, and assisting consumers and families through dental health education, and overcoming barriers to consistent ongoing care (Petrosky, Shaffter, Devlin, & Almog, 2000).

Because of the rapid recent transformation of health care, it might be assumed that social work in community health is a new invention. However, nothing could be further from the truth, as a brief overview of the history of social work in health care demonstrates.

A Brief History of Social Work in Health Care

Medical social work was one of the first areas of practice and the first specialization to occur in the profession. The initial development of medical social work was closely linked to hospitals and physicians. By the mid–nineteenth century, volunteers and paid employees provided home visits to new mothers and their infants to assess the multiple social and environmental conditions that might lead to infant mortality. These efforts initiated what the profession has since referred to as the casework method. In 1907, the Charity Organization Societies (COS) and Johns Hopkins Medical School joined forces to provide medical students with first-hand experience of the social and environmental factors that might affect their patients. In order to accomplish that objective, social workers—known as caseworkers—took medical students into the inner city neighborhoods of Baltimore on patient home visits (Rudolph, 2000). The purpose of this innovation was to afford the physician—who otherwise did not know of the patient's home life or circumstances—with experiential knowledge of the social and psychological aspects of the patient's life.

At about the same period, Dr. Richard Cabot of Massachusetts General Hospital, Boston, sought to combine social work and medical care leading to the initial legitimization of social work as an entity in hospitals. At the time, medical care was also undergoing a transformation (Starr, 1982). That is, health care delivery was moving from the tradition of physicians making home visits to deliver care, to patients visiting physicians in their offices in order to receive care. Thus, the social work role "linked" the physician with the patient's social and family world by providing the physician with that knowledge. In 1918, indicative of the development of social work in health care and the expanding field of medicine, the first professional social work organization, the American Association of Hospital Social Workers, formalized the profession of health care social work (Rudolph, 2000; Volland, 1996). Spurred by the public health movement and the social problems associated with increasing numbers of immigrant and poor populations, social workers were leaders in community and population specific health care efforts. Jane Addams's work exemplifies community-based social work that focused largely on the interdependence of the health of individuals, families, and their communities, and in orchestrating a psychosocial perspective in the sanitation movement.

In the decades that followed, social workers were integral in developing health care programs in the settlement house movement, maternal-child health, and in practice that connected health with social care, especially for the poor. These social movements and accomplishments led social workers into the specialty known then as public health social work. In the mid-1930s, the national movement promoting the health of children and mothers as a social value was spearheaded by social workers, such as Julia Lathrop, director of the Children's Bureau, resulting in the first national prioritizing of prenatal and child health care. Linking health care consumers and their environments with physicians and health care systems is a theme that spans decades of health care social work, built the foundation of the person-in-the-environment perspective, and set the profession apart from nurses and physicians early in the history of the health care professions in the United States.

By the 1950s medical social workers were, however, in practice largely inside hospitals making referrals to the community, but rarely being active in the community. Health care social work transitioned from community-centered to hospital-centered practice and to centering on patients' intrapsychic issues, rather than their psychosocial-environmental contexts. Not surprisingly, hospital social workers adopted the medical model of diagnosis and treatment; a patient and his or her current illness is an "event," and care is a three-part sequence relating to that event only: hospitalization, medical intervention(s), and discharge. Social work's role in health care identified primarily, if not solely, with the latter part of the sequence. Thus, over the next several decades, in consort with efforts to control hospital costs, social work practice in health care was limited, and some would say sequestered, to the role of discharge planner in hospitals. More recently the focus on community health and evidence of the relationships between physical illness, psychosocial, behavioral, and cultural issues prompt attention to social work in ambulatory health care practice (Institute of Medicine, 2001).

In summary, social work in health care is a century-old field of professional practice. The paradigm shift in health care delivery of recent years generates opportunities in new areas for practice and addresses the health needs of vulnerable populations. Parallel to these opportunities is the challenge to meet the needs of diverse consumer populations, and to respond effectively to the mandates for evidenced-based, time-limited interventions.

Social Work Practice in Community-Based Health Care in the Twenty-First Century

By the beginning of the twenty-first century, accumulating evidence substantiated the connections between economic poverty, such as in many inner city and rural areas, and limited educational and social resources, physical health, major health risks, and the etiology of several diseases (Feldman, 2001; Institute of Medicine, 2001). The door was open for social work to move outside the hospital and reach, once again, into the ecological, biopsychosocial, and community environment of health care practice in a variety of new settings, or as Rosenberg and Holden (1997) suggest to return to Hull House and COS traditions.

Social work practice in the current world of community health requires a combination of direct and indirect knowledge and skills. In summary, social work practice in community-based health care necessitates an integration of

- knowledge of culture/cultural background; major disease conditions, especially in at-risk populations; consumer population trends; community-based interdisciplinary health care program development and implementation; and prevention;
- expertise in interdisciplinary health care communication; teams and collaboration; advanced information technologies; evidence-based, time-limited, culturally competent assessment and interventions; care coordination; community program planning and implementation; and practice and program evaluation.

SETTINGS FOR SOCIAL WORK PRACTICE IN AMBULATORY COMMUNITY HEALTH CARE

First, some discussion of the nature of community health care settings for social work is warranted. Ambulatory health care settings are generally host settings for social work. Host settings are characteristically organizations and agencies dominated by professions, authority, decision making, and management other than social work—characteristics that have implications for social work practice (Gibelman, 2003). The next section of this chapter explores social work roles, practice, interdisciplinary collaboration, and teamwork in several host settings in ambulatory health, including

- primary care,
- faith-based health care organizations,
- multiple organization/community partnerships.

Later chapters focus on practice with individual consumers and their families and on behalf of consumer populations.

Primary Care

Social work in primary care, though not new in the United States, is an expanding area for practice having a somewhat longer history in Britain (Lymberry & Milward, 2001; Rock & Cooper, 2000). Primary care is defined by the Institute of Medicine (1994) as the health consumer's physician-centered first point of contact with a health care system that provides ongoing management of new and old health problems, identifies and coordinates specialty care providers, and delivers comprehensive services, particularly as related to preventive health care. Primary care is intended to promote physical, mental, and psychosocial health by integrating and providing services (Cowles, 2003). The extent of psychosocial needs of health consumers is suggested by estimates that one-quarter of general medicine patients, and up to one-half of poor, uninsured primary care patients, have a mental illness (Mauksch et al., 2001; Olfson et al., 2000; Rock & Cooper, 2000). It is also of note that the physician as primary care provider is a role amenable to managed care and its identification of the physician as gatekeeper to all services for patients (Van Hook, 2003).

The center of primary care is an ongoing, trusting relationship between patients and their physicians. Research findings suggest that a strong relationship with a primary care provider enhances patient satisfaction, improves preventive care, and may lower health care costs (Bindman, Grumbach, Osmond, Vranizan, & Stewart, 1996; Kao, Green, Zaslavsky, Koplan, & Cleary, 1998; Weiss & Blustein, 1996). Conversely, communication barriers are detrimental to the formation of a trusting relationship and effective care (e.g., Schilder, Kennedy, Goldstone, Ogden, Hogg, & O'Shaugnessy, 2001; Weiss & Blustein, 1996). A trusting relationship with health care providers may be particularly important for patients from populations who are at risk for illness or in poor health due to ecological, social, and/or economic disadvantage.

Patients with complex psychosocial needs may make heavy demands on primary care providers (Berkman et al., 1996; Lesser, 2000). Research findings suggest that about one-half of consumers may first seek care for psychosocial problems in primary care settings (Badger, Ackerson, Buttell, & Rand, 1997). Psychosocial problems include concrete issues, such as employment, family problems, and mental health issues, including depression and anxiety, and so on. For instance, Van Hook (2003) reports that three-quarters (76 percent) of the primary care patients in her study ($n = 229$) were assessed by their social worker with family problems and over one-half (55 percent) with depression.

However, physicians, due to the time constraints and the absence of psychosocial content in their traditional medical training, may overlook their patients' psychosocial problems and have difficulty discussing these problems with consumers (Brook, Gordon, Meadow & Cohen, 2000; DeCoster & Egan, 2001; Simonian & Tarnowski, 2001). Thus, primary physicians can benefit from the knowledge and skills that social workers bring to primary care (Lesser, 2000; Netting & Williams, 2000). A team approach by primary care physicians and social workers facilitates a continuity of care and services for patients with multiple psychosocial and health problems and supports physicians' care. Some suggest that patients may well accept social work services available within primary care when they would not otherwise seek these services (e.g., Badger, Ackerson, Buttell, & Rand, 1997).

Primary care endorses disease management. Disease management is an empirically validated, interdisciplinary intervention model that has gained the attention of managed care (Claiborne & Vandenburgh, 2001; Hunter & Fairfield, 1997). Disease management reflects some of the principles of behavioral medicine. Behavioral medicine incorporates consumers' psychosocial issues and health conditions, and it seeks to improve health by controlling or reducing the extent of negative effects of a medical condition (Brook, Gordon, Meadow, & Cohen, 2000).

As an example of effectiveness of the disease management, Steinman and colleagues (2003) report significantly improved quality of life, cost savings, and glycemic control (i.e., control of blood sugar levels) in a disease management program with diabetic geriatric patients (Steinman, Steinman, & Steinman, 2003). As a second example, evaluation of an innovative project placing a disease management program for children with asthma and their families in a school setting found significant health outcome improvements (Tinkelman & Schwartz, 2004) including

- significant decreases in the children's asthmatic symptoms and attacks and in school absences due to asthma;
- significant increases in knowledge of asthma, asthma attack triggers, and medication use for both the children and their family caregivers;
- significantly improved quality of life of family caregivers.

Social Work Practice in Primary Care Settings

Social work practice in primary care is heterogeneous because the settings in which it occurs are highly varied. For instance, primary care can occur in single or group practice physicians' offices, health department clinics, or faith-based programs. Much of the literature on social work in primary care to date focuses somewhat narrowly on social workers providing mental health services in physicians' offices. In comparison, family practice, a relative new field of medical practice, is an example of a primary care setting identified recently as having multiple possibilities and advantages for social work in addition to mental health services (Lesser, 2000).

In general, the social worker in primary health care settings is responsible for psychosocial services including efficient assessment and time-limited interventions for a wide range of illness-related problems and needs, and coordinating care and services. These practice activities help ensure a continuity of care, can prevent medical crises, and improve efficiency in care provision. Practices that target health-related behavioral change, promote health, and are empirically evaluated, such as disease management and cognitive behavioral individual and group interventions, are highly pertinent to social work practice in primary care settings (Claiborne & Vandenburgh, 2001; Comer, 2004; Harris & Franklin, 2003). A second area of social work practice in primary care is consultation and education with physicians, other providers, and staff. Consultation might concern the psychosocial aspects of an individual patient's medical condition or appropriate psychosocial interventions, or topics of concern for groups of consumers.

Interdisciplinary collaboration is an essential component of primary care, especially for practice with at-risk, vulnerable, and disadvantaged consumer populations, such as the aging, low-income prenatal/postnatal patients, or the underinsured/uninsured (Cameron & Mauskch, 2002; Scholle & Kelleher, 1999). In host settings, social workers' collaborative skills are indispensable for effective practice and positive patient outcomes. Collaboration models range from minimal to full integration of social workers and physicians and other providers (Lesser, 2000). In the minimal, or corollary model, physicians may refer to social workers patient by patient, just as they refer to other professionals. In the integrated model, social workers collaborate as partners with physicians and other disciplines. In primary care settings, the integrated collaboration model is endorsed over the former model (Lesser, 2000; Nettings & Williams, 2000; Rock & Cooper, 2000).

Research findings on primary care physicians' views of collaboration with social workers are inconsistent. Some findings reflect the corollary model of collaboration; physicians describe a role for social workers reminiscent of discharge planning in hospitals, such as facilitating nursing home placement, determining eligibility for coverage, and coordinating community referrals (Badger, Ackerson, Buttell, & Rand, 1997). Others describe social workers as the "eyes and ears" of primary care physicians, a description that is closer to the integrated model of social worker–physician collaboration (Netting & Williams, 2000, p. 237).

Family health community centers, a variant of primary care, may be the next evolution in health care delivery and a venue for providing social work in community-based health care (Cameron & Mauskch, 2002). Family health centers provide comprehensive health services to consumers with a variety of health concerns in a particular neighborhood, community, or geographic area. The centers may be located in public schools, churches, community, or neighborhood centers. These centers may have a single focus, delivering only one type of health care, or a wide spectrum of health, social, and mental health services. Social work practice in family health centers is similar to practice in traditional primary care in that it may include assessment and short-term problem-solving counseling, but often also incorporates health education, wellness, and disease management programs for consumers, their families, and community members.

In summary, social work in primary care or family health centers involves a range of practice activities spanning direct services with individual consumers, groups of consumers, interdisciplinary collaboration, interdisciplinary education, coordination of services, health promotion, and wellness programs.

Ethical Issues in Primary Care Settings

Inclusion of social work in the traditional physician-patient relationship in primary health care settings can enhance consumer well-being and continuity of care, but may also result in ethical difficulties for social workers given the profession's ethical commitment to patient well-being, confidentiality, and/or self-determination. By way of illustration, social work practice in primary care settings includes the possibility that a consumer's needs for care may exceed the extent of care allowed by the managed care plan. This situation presents an ethical conflict for social workers because of ethical obligations to the well-being of both their clients and employing organization. Professional ethical commitments to client confidentiality and to quality of care may conflict when a consumer identifies problems with the medical care provided or with the primary care physician to the social worker (Congress, 1999; Lesser, 2000; Rock & Congress, 1999). Cross-cultural issues may further complicate the issues with potential ethical conflicts over client self-determination, when the consumer and the physician or other providers do not share a common view of Western medical care, or when consumers distrust providers who are not of their own culture.

Social Work in Faith-Based Health Care

Pro-social principles and faith-related programs were hallmarks of early social work health care efforts in the last century. With recent legislation opening access to government funding and increasing political and public acceptance of faith-based social and health programs, faith-based programs have multiplied.

Social work practice in faith-based community health programs calls for some specific areas of knowledge in addition to those noted previously in this chapter. Clear knowledge of the funding capacities of Charitable Choice legislation and the restrictions on funded organizations is essential. Social work knowledge of program planning and development is important in FBOs that receive funds through Charitable Choice venues or by direct congregational support. Knowledge and skills in leadership to address potential value conflicts between providers, staff, and health care consumers are pertinent to social work practice in these settings. Understanding the interactions of cultural background elements, in particular those associated with spiritual orientation and health beliefs, are value-added attributes for social workers in FBO ambulatory health care settings.

Given the social and political positions of some faith and religious organizations, value conflicts between FBO providers and health care consumers are possible. For social workers, these value conflicts may constitute professional ethical dilemmas. For example, because Charitable Choice policies restrict recipients from using funds for religious instruction of consumers, striking the balance between faith-based environments and imposing faith-related expectations on consumers might be challenging in light of the profession's ethical commitment to consumer self-determination. In illustration, social workers in faith-based health care programs can be instrumental in assuring access to care for consumers who have lifestyles or needs, such as consumers who are gay, seek family planning, or are pregnant and single, that may conflict with the values of a faith organization. Social work expertise in advocacy, negotiating conflicts, and teamwork is invaluable to assure access to needed health care in these instances.

Partnerships, Health Promotion, and Prevention in Community Health Care

Partnerships, whether between universities and community organizations or among community organizations, seek in general to resolve health care problems of fragmentation and/or limited resources. The objectives of these partnerships may be

- coordination of health care delivery for specific at-risk or vulnerable consumers across multiple organizations to resolve gaps in services;

- creation of formal infrastructures to integrate the service delivery of multiple provider organizations.

The latter objective—the creation of formal infrastructures—is designed to resolve fragmentation of resources and services by developing mechanisms and programs that integrate services of multiple, but disconnected, providers and/or agencies who share a consumer population or target the same health condition. Social workers in community/organizational partnerships possess multiple professional skills and contribute to areas of knowledge including

- community or population needs assessment;
- program planning, development, and implementation;
- interorganizational collaboration and community coalitions.

Social workers' skills for building collective strengths and relationships and negotiating conflicts among groups are integral to developing community health programs for culturally diverse consumer populations, groups, and organizations.

An example of a university-community partnership in health care is a program to provide services in schools for asthmatic, inner city children (Mosley, 1998). The purpose of the neighborhood-based Baltimore program—an initiative of Johns Hopkins Community Health Institute—was to provide a seamless delivery system for children with asthma in four public schools to improve

- children's access to medical care;
- children's access to pharmaceuticals;
- links between the school-based program and the children's neighborhoods.

The partnership, led and staffed by social workers, involved a spectrum of stakeholders including university faculty, the elementary school children and their parents, school personnel, school nurses, local business owners, social service agency representatives, and managed care organizations serving the geographic area.

Prevention and Health Promotion

In the aggregate, the shift to community-based care, programs focusing on specific disease(s) or population(s), primary care, family health centers, disease management protocols, and priorities of managed care give impetus to increasing attention to prevention and health promotion. Thus, an overview of the perspective and a brief discussion of prevention are pertinent.

Public health and the biomedical model differ to some degree in their explanations of illness. From the public health viewpoint, illness is caused by multiple societal (e.g., sanitation, education about health, infrastructure adequacy) and biological (e.g., control of communicable diseases) factors. The purpose of public health is the protection and improvement of community health for a population, designated by commonly held demographics, characteristics, or geography, through organized community-based efforts by

- the prevention of factors that lead to ill health;
- the promotion of factors that lead to better health or reduce risk factors.

There are three categories of prevention: primary, secondary, and tertiary. The purpose of primary prevention programs is to reduce the susceptibility to disease or illness or the social problems of at-risk individuals or populations. Education efforts regarding the dangers of smoking or unsafe sex, including those educating a community in general and those targeting at-risk populations, exemplify primary prevention. The goal of secondary prevention programs is the early detection of diseases or illnesses so that interventions to change behaviors and/or risk factors can prevent the irreversible negative consequences of the disease or illness. Screening programs for hypertension, breast cancer, and diabetes are examples of secondary prevention efforts. The focus of tertiary prevention programs is to ameliorate the consequences of disease(s) or illness(es) by assisting consumers in the management of existing conditions. This level of prevention is the most familiar to health care social workers because it reflects generalist practice activities, such as care coordination, discharge planning, locating and coordinating concrete and service resources.

Any of the three levels of prevention may programmatically target a single disease, such as asthma, or a particular population, such as teenage mothers, or a more general population, such as women. In any case, programs might occur through a single organization, or through a network of connected organizations or agencies.

Health promotion is a particular approach in primary prevention. Health promotion addresses social and environmental factors that contribute to disease, such as a lack of knowledge, and often utilizes empowerment. For instance, Auslander and colleagues report the efficacy of a community-based health promotion program for low-income African-American women at risk for diabetes that incorporated peer, rather than professional, educators and leaders (Auslander, Haire-Joshu, Houston, Rhee, & Williams, 2002). The specifics of health promotion are discussed in Chapter 5 on direct practice and Chapter 6 on practice on behalf of consumer populations.

ADVANCES IN COMMUNICATION TECHNOLOGY FOR HEALTH CARE PRACTICE

The use of what was once termed "telemedicine" and is now, because the scope of the use of telecommunication technology is expansive, known as telehealth is rapidly expanding because of advances in the technologies themselves, the creative efforts of health care professionals, and increases in funding from third party payers and the government. For example, recent legislation—Improvement and Protection Act of 2000—expanded coverage for direct health care and services provided through telehealth technologies (Clemmitt, 2001).

For starters, the availability of Web-based health care information is growing by the second. This is a worthwhile avenue for consumers who may be isolated geographically or who, by virtue of having a comparatively rare condition, do not have access to care, social resources, and peers. The Pew Charitable Trust funded project on the Internet and American Life reports that 80 percent of Internet users (i.e., 93 million persons) use the Web to obtain health and medical information; three-quarters of those reported that their information about health improved, and many indicated that the information influenced their health care decisions (Pew Internet and American Life Project, 2000). Specialized Web sites offer information on specific diseases adapted to particular age and cultural groups; some Web sites include interactive programming. These resources are invaluable for practitioners and consumers, though some critical assessment is required to assure the quality of sites (see Appendix B on Web site summaries).

Telecommunication technologies are now available that can provide interactive direct contact between providers and consumers, and among consumers, without restrictions of geographical distance. Interactive health communication is the utilization of electronic communication technology or devices with consumers, or their caregivers, and health professionals to provide access to health care or address health-related concerns, the latter including support and information. For example, Farmer and Muhlenbruck (2001) describe telehealth direct service programs for largely rural children with special needs in seven states. Health care teams composed of physicians, nurses, social workers, psychologists, and physical, occupational, and speech therapists connect with the children and their families via videoconferencing to assess specific disorders (e.g., cerebral palsy, autism), to address primary care health issues (e.g., acute illness, wellness) and to provide treatment for emotional, social, and/or behavioral concerns.

As another illustration of the use of technology in practice, Heckman and colleagues (1999) describe a program to enhance the coping capacities of rural HIV+/AIDS consumers through telephone conference call delivered interventions (Heckman et al., 1999). The conceptual basis of the intervention package was cognitive appraisal of stress and coping in eight one-hour structured sessions that

- identified consumer stressors and coping resources;
- taught problem-solving and coping strategies;
- employed between session homework assignments.

Though the use of technology to deliver care is comparatively new, evaluation studies report positive outcomes (e.g., Farmer & Muhlenbruck, 2001; Piette, Kraemer, Weinberger, & McPhee, 2001).

Some technological advances have direct implications for social work practice. One example is the very recent revolution in genetics spearheaded by the Human Genome Project that produced the technology to identify probabilistic risk for some acute, potentially terminal, and/or debilitating chronic diseases. Identification of predisposing, risk, and carrier factors for several genetic disorders (e.g., Huntington's, sickle cell, cystic fibrosis, Tay-Sachs, breast and colon cancers) is now possible (National Human Genome Research Institute, 2005).

As a result of the information obtained through genetic testing, consumers may face multiple and often difficult decisions. When genetic testing identifies predisposing genetic factors, consumers can experience emotion-laden decisions about whether to inform family members of possible genetic predispositions; if so decided, they face further decisions concerning how and when to tell. Informing family members of genetic testing results can lead to their having to decide whether they themselves, too, want to be tested. On the other hand, early identification of such genetic risk factors does enable persons to modify psychosocial behaviors that would otherwise increase risk for disease, and to utilize early screening technology and interventions. The psychosocial stress of testing and subsequent decision making can be high; the support and guidance of skilled and knowledgeable social workers is important. Ethical considerations include confidentiality and access to results, including managed care and family members (Lowenberg, Dolgoff, & Harrington, 2000).

For example, genetic research has identified two genes, BRCA1 and BRCA2, that when transmitted in an altered (i.e., mutated) form are associated with an on average probabilistic increased risk of developing breast cancer by age seventy. Two in-depth research studies (Freedman, 1998; Oktay, 2005) found that genetic testing for breast cancer does not necessarily resolve ambiguous or complex health care decisions. On the one hand, even when the genetic test is negative, women's fears for their mothers, sisters, and nieces may continue. Often women who know that breast cancer occurred in their family may resist testing, while their mothers may strongly encourage it. For others, requests for testing are prompted to inform other medical decisions (e.g., whether to become pregnant, to have a prophylactic mastectomy, etc.). The advances in genetic testing illustrates poignantly that, while medical technology research has sped forward with amazing results, psychosocial research on humans experiencing these technologies has not (see Appendix B on Web site summaries for sites to obtain more information).

Technological advances in medicine also produce devices to assist consumers with particular health conditions. For example, devices are available for persons with diabetes that avoid painful daily needle sticks to measure blood sugar levels, some of which are programmable to monitor blood sugar, diet, and exercise. Computerized pumps the size of a pager can deliver insulin without injection. Another amazing advance in telecommunication technology is for individuals with Lou Gehrig's disease, a rapidly advancing neurological disease most often affecting adults in their thirties or forties that does not affect cognitive functioning, but culminates with total physical impairment including speech. Telecommunication incorporated with computer technology allows those with this devastating disease to record communications in their own voice, before the loss of speech. The ability to speak with family for these patients is a tremendous help in dealing with this devastating illness (see Appendix B on Web site summaries for sites to obtain more information).

In brief, technological advances in medicine have psychosocial ramifications for consumers and for practitioners. For consumers, these advances can predict or transform devastating illnesses to conditions that, though they may be long term or chronic, can be managed, albeit requiring lifestyle and psychosocial changes for the consumer and family. Advances in technologies require that practitioners continually acquire new knowledge, expertise, and critically analyze how to incorporate these advances in practice, and how the advances affect the psychosocial well-being and needs of consumers.

SUMMARY

So, what is social work practice in community-based health care? To the extent that roles can define practice, social work in community-based health is practice of a different sort. In brief, practice occurs in community settings, in either direct or indirect practice; in either case practice focuses on health care for at-risk consumer populations and on resolving unmet needs and the fragmentation of health care delivery. The chapter explored emerging settings and approaches for social work practice in ambulatory health care, including primary care, family health, faith-based health centers, and the emphasis on disease management and interdisciplinary practice in collaboration and teams. Advances in technologies, both medical and communication, health promotion, and prevention expand the practitioner's repertoire of resources for health care practice. In conclusion, ambulatory health care practice might be described as a return to the early history of social work in health as it responds to the needs of culturally diverse and vulnerable individuals, groups, and populations of consumers.

DISCUSSION QUESTIONS AND ACTIVITIES FOR INDIVIDUALS AND SMALL GROUPS

1. Explore each of the Web sites on genetics summarized in Appendix B of this text to gain knowledge about the testing, its use, and the advances in the Human Genome Project. What is your personal reaction to the advancing technologies? What are the challenges you might experience were you to have a consumer requesting genetic testing? How do you see yourself as a professional social worker addressing the potential for differential access to the technologies by minorities?
2. In reference to the content of this chapter on the emerging areas for social work practice, describe what is for you the perfect job, setting, and role in ambulatory health care practice.

GLOSSARY

advocacy: Practice activities targeted at educating, informing, or representing the needs and wishes of individuals, families, groups, and communities through direct interventions for client(s) or indirectly on behalf of groups of clients or populations.

Charity Organization Societies (COS): Private or philanthropically funded organization that delivered services to the poor, disenfranchised, or needy populations; workers were called friendly visitors.

disease management: A model of integrated, interdisciplinary care utilizing standardized medical protocols for specific diseases, emphasizing medical outcomes and evidence of effectiveness.

host setting: Organizations and agencies dominated by professions, authority, decision making, and management other than social work.

infant mortality: The proportion of newborns who die before their twenty-eighth day after birth; generally the proportion per 1,000 live births.

interdisciplinary: The process of professionals from various disciplines working together to provide integrated care to benefit the consumer or consumers.

multidisciplinary: The process of providing care from disciplines working side by side, or in parallel fashion, without integrating the plan of care for a consumer or consumers.

primary care: A medical approach in providing health care that manages, integrates, and coordinates services and providers through comprehensive and preventive health care.

primary prevention: The area of prevention activities that seeks to reduce the susceptibility to disease or illness or the social problems of individuals or populations.

public health: The art and science that deals with the protection and improvement of community health by organized community-based efforts.

secondary prevention: Prevention programs that target early detection of diseases or illnesses so that interventions to change behaviors or risk factors may be utilized before irreversible negative consequences of the disease or illness occur.

tertiary prevention: The area of preventive activities that seeks to manage an existing disease or illness in order to ameliorate negative consequences of the disease or illness.

wellness: The quality or state of being in good health, especially as an actively sought goal.

PART II:
CULTURALLY RESPONSIVE PRACTICE IN AMBULATORY HEALTH CARE

Chapter 5

Direct Practice in Community-Based Health Care

- *What is the focus of assessment in ambulatory health care?*
- *How can practitioners conceptualize practice?*
- *What is logic modeling and how does it guide planning?*
- *What is culturally responsive engagement? Assessment?*
- *What culturally responsive, evidence-based interventions are appropriate?*
- *How can social workers be effective in interdisciplinary teamwork?*
- *What is best practice in coordinating consumer care?*

INTRODUCTION

Previous chapters identified the knowledge and skills required for direct practice with ambulatory health care consumers. Briefly, community-based health care calls for practitioners who are proficient in ethically based, efficacious, time-limited, and culturally responsive engagement, assessment, and intervention, and in interdisciplinary teamwork in a variety of settings. Therefore, this chapter first presents a conceptual process and a technique for critical thinking, and relevant theories and concepts, followed by engaging and assessing consumers, selected time-limited evidence-based interventions, coordination of client care, and interdisciplinary team participation in culturally responsive direct practice. Related ethical considerations are included throughout the chapter.

The premise of each of these discussions is that the central focus of direct practice in ambulatory community-based health care is on the present health condition, and related consumer needs and concerns. The major direct practice task for social workers is ameliorating or resolving the psychosocial problems that result from chronic and new medical conditions, and challenge consumer well-being.

A CONCEPTUAL PROCESS AND A TECHNIQUE FOR CRITICAL THINKING

The time-limited nature of community health care social work requires efficiently planned assessment and intervention. Planning negates both random and habituated approaches to practice. Habituated approaches refer to workers implementing interventions routinely or by virtue of what an agency "just does," rather than critically analyzing and linking interventions to identified problems, theories, concepts, and empirical research (Gambrill, 1997). The first step is a conceptual process for direct practice.

A conceptual process guides the practitioner's thinking in understanding clients' current situations, health problems, and concerns, and in linking problems to be resolved with interventions. Figure 5.1 depicts a critical thinking process linking concepts and theories with consumer's issues, with interventions, and ultimately to evaluation.

Logic Modeling: A Technique and Tool for Planning Practice

The process shown in Figure 5.1 illustrates the process of linking concepts and theories in thinking through assessment and intervention with consumers. Logic modeling is a tool that provides a conceptual map for linking problems and interventions (Alter & Egan, 1997). A logic model leads to clear and comprehensive planning through the following components:

- problem and goal statements;
- a breakdown of the problem statement into a problem list and the goal statement into a list of objectives, or mini-goals, for each problem;
- identification of methods/interventions for each problem and objective;
- a list of the resources (inputs) needed to implement each of those methods.

Logic modeling begins with a narrative description of the situation the consumer is currently experiencing (i.e., the problem statement), which is then broken down into a problem list of specific issues. Next, the situation as it is expected to be after intervention is described (i.e., goal statement); this statement is then parsed into a list of objectives specifically linked to each problem. The methods/interventions section identifies the interventions or processes used for each problem to result in the related objective. The components of a logic model are depicted in Figure 5.2; arrows indicate the recursive linkages between components.

In this chapter, logic modeling collaboratively operationalizes the work to be done with a consumer. Logic modeling for programs on

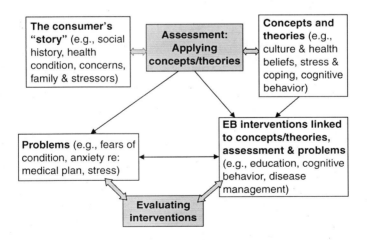

FIGURE 5.1. Assessment: Linking a consumer's story to theories/concepts, problems, interventions, and evaluation.

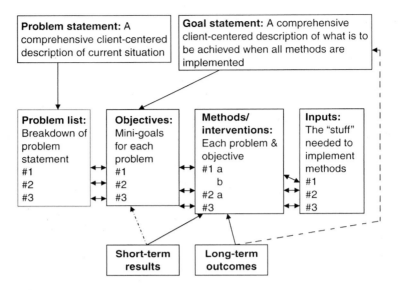

FIGURE 5.2. The components of a logic model.

behalf of populations of consumers is incorporated in the next chapter (Chapter 6).

PERSPECTIVES, CONCEPTS, AND THEORIES FOR DIRECT PRACTICE

Perspectives, concepts, and theories applicable to ambulatory health practice are the strengths perspective, ecological/family systems, stress and coping, and cognitive-behavioral theory. These concepts and theories are appropriate for practice in ambulatory health practice because they

- direct attention to a consumer's capacities, support, and resources;
- situate consumers and families socially and culturally;
- are pertinent to evidence-based practice.

Though it is beyond the scope of this text to detail each of these theories and concepts, a brief discussion of each is pertinent.

The Strengths and Ecological Perspectives

Viewing a consumer through the strengths perspective lens acknowledges that consumers have capacities they bring to the experience of having a medical condition, or diagnosis (Corwin, 2002). The perspective suggests that tapping into a client's usual coping strategies facilitates successful adjusting to an illness or health problem. On the other hand, based on the premise that they have successfully coped in the past, consumers facing a new medical situation may need to learn new coping skills, but have the capacity to do so. In either instance, the present health condition(s) will interact with the consumer's and family's cultural background, psychosocial capacities, and resources, as well as stressors that may exist in addition to the current illness. The strengths perspective directs the practitioner to consider the resources, capacities, and stressors of the client's ecological and family systems.

Corwin (2002) incorporates the strengths perspective and ecological systems concepts when she suggests that success or failure in adapting to a stressor is a function of the "severity and duration" of the stress (p. 25) and personal factors (e.g., resilience, temperament, life development, family/kinship support, etc.). The ecological and family systems viewpoint expands the practitioner's perspective beyond just the individual to the social relationships within which the individual is embedded. Relationships within systems bring both resources and stresses to members of the system. Ecological and family systems contribute to the self-identify of individuals, and interact with the cultural background(s) of the family, the social network, and community.

Stress Appraisal and Coping Theory

A diagnosis of a long-term or life-altering health condition, such as hypertension, or extensive medical care, such as strict diet regimens, or lifestyle changes are likely to cause some level of stress. According to this theory, an individual's response to experience(s) is a function of appraising (i.e., evaluating) both the stress and the ability to cope with the stress (Lazarus & Folkman, 1984). In brief, the individual appraises the stress ("How bad is this?"), and their abilities/capacities to cope with that stress ("Do I know how to deal with this?

How well can I deal with this?"). In brief, a consumer's evaluation of coping capacity includes assessing past coping strategies and applying these to the current situation, and resources. In practice, the theory's utility is that it directs the ambulatory health care practitioner's attention to assess a consumer's stress reaction to current health conditions or problems and to the consumer's coping capacities.

Cognitive-Behavioral Theory

Cognitive-behavioral theory is pertinent in community health because interventions derived from the theory are both evidence based and time limited (Comer, 2004; Dziegielewski & Holliman, 2001; Ligon, 1998). This theory suggests that thinking (i.e., cognition) determines behavior and feelings (Beck, 1995; Hepworth, Rooney, & Larsen, 2002). Thinking is conceptually defined as the messages, or statements, that we say to ourselves ("self-talk"); patterns of thinking are referred to as schema. Schema may be functional and lead to successful, adaptive behaviors and positive feelings or be irrational and illogical leading to behavioral problems and negative feelings. Cognitive-behavioral concepts direct the practitioner's attention to a consumer's thinking patterns about an illness or medical treatments.

In brief, the ecological and strengths perspectives, stress and coping theory, and cognitive-behavioral theory guide thinking about the issues of concern to health care consumers and interventions. Logic modeling specifies problems, objectives to be achieved, and the relationships between assessed problems and interventions.

CULTURALLY RESPONSIVE PRACTICE

Engagement and Forming an Alliance

Given the time-limited nature of practice in community-based health, consulting with interdisciplinary team members before the initial meeting is important as it can provide necessary information (i.e., health care coverage, medical conditions, planned or current medical interventions, cultural background) that can sharpen the focus of the initial contact with clients. Having this information also lessens the possibility of redundant questions, communicates coherence among interdisciplinary providers, and attends to the effective use of limited time.

Effective direct practice in community-based health care, as in all other areas of direct practice, begins with effective engagement. Engagement is the process of establishing a relationship (i.e., alliance) between the practitioner and the consumer/consumer family. The result of effective engagement is a positive working alliance, which is a requisite to effective assessment and intervention. Building rapport, infusing a sense of optimism, and joining in a consumer-centered process promotes a positive alliance. In the time-limited nature of practice in ambulatory health practice, engaging and forming a positive alliance needs to occur rapidly. Corwin (2002) recommends beginning the alliance and the focus of practice during the first phone call or meeting. Workers can foster an effective alliance by explaining their role, and clarifying the consumer's understanding of the reasons for and expectations about the purpose of meeting together.

Given the emphasis on short-term treatment, the practitioner must accomplish several objectives in the first session. Flexibility regarding the length of this session is an advantage because the number of sessions may be limited. Boyd-Franklin (2003) urges practitioners to see establishing trust with black clients as their first task; reaching out directly to new clients is recommended as is conveying respect because African Americans are often reluctant to use social work services. Practitioners can consider sharing some personal background particularly with clients from cultures whose worldview is based on and values personal connections, such as Latinos, to build rapport and smooth the progress of engagement. Engaging and forming an effective working alliance with culturally diverse consumers is promoted when the practitioner takes on the inquiring stance of a learner concerning the consumer's cultural background; listens with interest; remains open-minded, nonjudgmental, and respectful of the consumer's cultural background; and paces communication to the conversational and cultural style of the client and/or family.

For example, exploration early in the process of an initial session about preferences for addressing consumers (e.g., Miss, Mrs., Mr.) or whether children should be spoken to directly is warranted, as is determining the appropriateness of shaking hands or other social touch and being cognizant of the culturally varying meanings attributed to gestures, eye contact, and physical proximity (Boyd-Franklin, 2003; Weaver, 2005). Practitioners who acknowledge their own sensitivity, but limited knowledge, of these possibilities are demonstrating their respect for consumers' cultural social rules and values and can facilitate establishing open communication in the worker-client relationship. Specific culturally related issues relevant to social worker–consumer/family interviews include expectations about promptness, or "clock time," and about initiating sessions with "small talk," or social chat.

Effective Communication with Consumers

Social workers utilize several generic techniques for effective communication in the engagement and the assessment process that are worth briefly reviewing considering the time-limited nature of practice. In brief review, these include facilitation (e.g., "Please do go on."); reflection (e.g., "It sounds like you think that . . . like you feel that . . ."); clarification (e.g., "Could you help me understand what you mean?"); confrontation (e.g., "You say you aren't afraid of [treatment], but you look fearful"); summarizing (e.g., organizing and summing up the discussion/interactions of the meeting).

Facilitating and reflecting comments helps build rapport and demonstrates that the practitioner is listening and nonjudgmental. Clarifying questions responds to the recommendation to take on a learner's stance with consumers of diverse backgrounds. Some caution is warranted regarding the use of confrontation in that the cultural background of some consumers may find its use invasive or rude (also see Chapter 3 on cultural competence).

Some communication styles controvert effective engagement and communication, such as avoidance and silence in response to a consumer verbalizing "unpleasant" feelings (e.g., anger) or topics (e.g., medication side effects on sexual functioning). Advising and using authority with consumers and/or their families distances the worker and can shut down open communication. An obvious consideration in engagement is the consumer's and worker's compatibility in language.

Brevity of contact in ambulatory health care necessitates that the practitioner is highly active and may be more directive. The practitioner's focus is on the here and now; identifying and enhancing the client/ client system's coping capacities with the present health condition is a primary objective. In this context, social workers might feel pressure to speed things along or focus on agency-required paperwork, thereby missing the opportunity afforded by the first contact to connect with consumers and families. It is just because of the time-pressured context of community health care settings that these initial moments are so important for effective practice. In summary, practitioners are focused and culturally responsive in the process of engagement and forming a positive alliance with consumers.

CULTURALLY RESPONSIVE ASSESSMENT

It is important to note that even in the time-limited context of managed care, assessment is not an event heralded by the completion of a form or forms, but a process. As depicted in Figure 5.1, the process of assessment reciprocally applies concepts and theories to the consumer's information and story. In ambulatory health care, assessment specifically includes exploring

- the influence of the current health condition(s) on the client's functioning and lifestyle;
- the consumer's concerns and questions about medical conditions and care;
- the consumer's capacities for coping with medical conditions and care.

Assessment is centered on the here and now, referencing to experiences in the past only to discern consumer's normal coping strategies, collecting information and synthesizing an understanding of the consumer's cultural background as it interfaces with the illness, and the receipt of health care from Western-model providers.

An initial meeting should conclude with worker and consumer/ family mutually agreeing on goals, targets for intervention, issues for next sessions, and contracting on those goals and issues. In a time-limited context, goals narrow the scope of the work to be done, are specific to the present health condition and its related stress, and must be achievable.

The Strengths of Culturally Diverse
Family Structures and Roles

When viewed through a culturally responsive lens and the strengths perspective, diverse family structures, patterns, and values are strengths, not problems to be solved, or barriers to positive inter-actions with professionals, or to positive health outcomes. Colleagues who are not trained in this perspective may benefit from practitioners reframing the structure, values, and health beliefs of culturally diverse consumers and families. For example, the presence of an extended or augmented family structure can be a support system for the client in adapting to the stress of a new diagnosis or an exacerbation of an existing illness. This reframe also evidences social work expertise for the team, and can result in better care planning and consumer-team interactions.

Culturally competent practitioners routinely include exploring family structure and roles by asking, for example, "Who is in your family, your household?" and "Who in the family makes health care decisions concerning family members?" Other possibilities of persons to consider in working with a consumer and family are church/mosque/temple "family" members and/or persons from the consumer's cultural community. In the health care context, practitioner's exploration of the consumer/family's understanding of the health condition and cause, acceptability of Western medicine, and use of cultural/folk/alternative health care and/or healer(s) is vital. With the information gained, the social worker can then consider whether there may be conflicts between the Western and ethnocultural medications or care a consumer uses. An inquiring stance as a learner lets the practitioner utilize such questions as these:

- "Might you help me understand how might someone with [client's cultural background] describe or understand your present health condition?"
- "Are their ways of treating your condition from your culture that you might use?"

A respectful inquiring stance in relation to spiritual orientation includes exploring how clients see their role with the current health issue(s), and whether their faith may be helpful in getting well. Discussion of prayer, meditation, or attendance in formal organizational or cultural community activities might begin by asking, "How do you and your family practice your faith or religion?" Understanding the connections of diverse consumers to local cultural communities, the extent of acceptance/acculturation to Western medicine, and immigration issues is very relevant.

Tools and Instruments for Assessment and Screening

The purpose of assessment and screening instruments is twofold:

- identifying needs;
- acquiring data for evaluation of practice.

Some assessment instruments only identify areas of need, while others accomplish that objective while also collecting data for evaluation of interventions.

Several psychosocial assessments are available in the literature, such as, among others, the Culturagram, family genograms and ecological system maps, and general assessment guides and, in addition, agency assessment forms (Boyd-Franklin, 2003; Congress, 2004; Hepworth, Rooney, & Larsen, 2002). Assessment tools can guide and foster consistency across assessments, and clarify areas for intervention. However, they do not measure levels of problems, identify issues needing further assessment, or furnish data for evaluation of the effectiveness of interventions.

The second purpose, as noted previously, is acquiring data for evaluating interventions. To fulfill that purpose, an instrument must result in data that indicate the degree or level of a psychosocial problem, be easy to use and to score, and preferentially are brief. Standardized instruments—ones with proven validity and reliability—are widely recommended as the profession pursues evidence-based practice.

A few valid and reliable assessment instruments are worthy of note: the SF-36 and its briefer forms, the Hudson Short-Form Assessment Scales, the Alcohol Use Disorders Identification Test (AUDIT), and the PSC. Each of these tools is briefly discussed in the following paragraphs.

Of particular utility in assessment and data collection in social work practice in community health settings are the SF-36 and its shorter forms, the SF-12, SF-8, and the SF-36 + Social Work (Berkman et al., 1999; Berkman & Marmaldi, 2001; Maramaldi, Berkman, & Barusch, 2005). The SF-36 scales screen health-related problems and mental illnesses. They measure how a health condition or disease may be affecting various domains of a consumer's life. The instruments link current health problems to limitations in physical activity, social activity, job performance, family relations, and energy levels, and general mental and emotional well-being. For instance, items ask the consumers how their present health condition has limited walking and climbing stairs; answer options are categorical from "yes, limited a lot" to "no, not at all limited." Items on emotional well-being relate, for example, to limitations due to the medical condition on the amount of time spent on work and are answered dichotomously (i.e., yes/no). Extent of emotions is tapped by items measuring how much of the time a client feels recently concerning, for example, nervousness or tiredness; each item is answered from "all" to "none" of the time. Maramaldi and coresearchers (2005) recently noted that the scales have not been validated across all cultures and, given the constructs the SF-36 measures, recommend that practitioners evaluate its appropriateness for culturally diverse consumers (Maramaldi, Berkman, & Barusch, 2005). The SF-36 is licensed and must be purchased.

The Hudson Short-Form Assessment Scales are widely validated instruments that assess several psychological and psychosocial factors of clients twelve years of age and older, have clinical cut-points, provide data for evaluation of interventions, and are available in Spanish. Clinical cut-points on each scale indicate scores above which intervention is indicated. The Hudson package includes scales measuring, for example, anxiety, stress, family relationships, depression, child behavior, and self-esteem measures (WALMYR Publishing, 2005). The scales are available in paper and computer-assisted format, each has twenty-five items, and each can be completed by the consumer in ten to twelve minutes by hand or with the computerized version; scoring is possible by hand or with the computerized program.

A recent meta-analysis of several instruments for screening of alcohol misuse that poses a risk for future problems reported that the Alcohol Use Disorders Identification Test (AUDIT) is the most widely validated alcohol screening tool, and this tool is sensitive for detecting alcohol misuse when used alone, or as part of a broader assessment (U.S. Preventive Services Task Force, 2004). The AUDIT is a ten-item scale; items measure the frequency and quantity of drinking by adults. As an example, items ask, "How many drinks containing alcohol do you have on a typical day?" and "How often during the last year have you had a feeling of guilt or remorse after drinking?" The AUDIT is easily scored and has a clinical cut-point of eight total points for the ten items indicating the likelihood of harmful alcohol use (U.S. Department of Health and Human Services, Substance Abuse and Mental Health Administration, National Clearinghouse of Alcohol and Drug Information, Substance Abuse, 2004). The AUDIT is available online and scoring procedures are included (see Appendix B on Web site summaries for sources of the SF-36, AUDIT, and Hudson scales).

Simonian and Tarnowski (2001) and others (Semansky, Koyanagi, & Vandivort-Warren, 2003) recommend the parent-completed PSC to screen for psychosocial problems in school-aged children and to identify children needing further assessment. Their research on the PSC produced clinical cut-points (i.e., scores above which further assessment and/or intervention is warranted). They suggest that the scale is sensitive to socioeconomic characteristics. The checklist is recommended in the evaluation of the federally mandated pediatric Early and Periodic Screening, Diagnosis, and Treatment (EPSDT) protocols.

Documentation in Health Settings

Documentation requirements are critically important to demonstrate the value of social work in care and to evidence HIPAA compliance (Kane, Houston-Vega, Tan, and Hawkins, 2002). The mandates of managed care require that the first session address and document coverage, coverage limits, consent forms, any relevant legalities (e.g., confidentiality, transmission of consumer information), personal financial resources, and the consumer's present medical/health condition(s). Documentation must include the specifics of HIPAA requirements, as detailed in Chapter 1. At a minimum, documentation must record client-worker contacts as evidence for coverage, and demonstrate ethical practice as protection against liability, and the relationship of social work interventions to the client's identified medical conditions.

An Application of Conceptually Assessing and the Logic Model Technique

An application of the conceptual process previously discussed for linking a consumer's story with theories and concepts in assessment discussed to this point is illustrative at this point. Let us suppose that a social worker in a primary health care setting is asked to see a consumer, Mrs. Thompson, and provided the following information:

> Mrs. Thompson is a forty-four-year-old African American diagnosed with hypertension and high cholesterol four months ago; she has health coverage. The physician notes that she is having difficulty in fulfilling her part of a disease management plan in making recommended lifestyle changes to increase physical activity and adhere to a nutrition plan.

In meeting with Mrs. Thompson, the practitioner finds that Mrs. Thompson's family includes a daughter and grandchild who live with her, two older daughters and their families who live in the city, and a son whom she rarely sees; the older daughters' father is deceased, and she rarely sees her younger daughter's and son's father, though she is very close to her own three siblings and their families. She is actively engaged in her church and is employed there as well. She is worried about her blood pressure, but feels God will take care. She does not see how she can "get active" since she works full time and takes care of her grandchild after work. As the primary cook, she wants to give the family good food—not what she is supposed to eat—and does not get to cooking that food for herself.

Stress appraisal and coping theory suggests that Mrs. Thompson's evaluation is that the stresses of lifestyle changes are beyond her coping capacities. Application of the ecological and strengths' perspectives identifies a sizable social and family system; however, some elements seem to take more support and care from Mrs. Thompson than they provide. Culturally related concepts suggest that her faith may have an influence on her health beliefs, is a major source of support, and is a coping mechanism for her. In brief, the concepts and assessment process of Mrs. Thompson's story highlight several concepts and theories that are explanatory in understanding her concerns and issues.

Mrs. Thompson's logic model would describe a problem statement inclusive of being overwhelmed by the stresses of family caregiving and work, resulting in difficulty in lifestyle changes and medical regimen adherence such that management of her hypertension and cholesterol levels is compromised. The problem list includes high stress levels from (1) multiple family responsibilities, (2) full-time work responsibilities, with (3) resultant difficulty in medical regimen compliance. Related objectives might include stress reduction, increased support for lifestyle changes, and weight and cholesterol level reductions.

In summary, culturally competent and effective engagement and communication is crucial in time-limited practice to forming a positive working alliance with consumers. Assessment incorporates exploration of cultural elements and focuses on the health issue at hand within the consumer's cultural, family, and social systems; the consumer's responses to the condition, capacities, and resources for achieving positive health outcomes; and acquiring data for evaluation with standardized measurements.

EVIDENCE-BASED INTERVENTIONS

Social work in ambulatory health care focuses on increasing consumers' abilities to cope with medical conditions, make lifestyle changes that enhance health, and overcome psychosocial barriers that might impede positive health outcomes. Because practice time may be limited, and substantiating the efficacy of interventions is required, best practice suggests the use of evidence-based interventions.

In addition, some techniques generic to practice are very relevant to time-limited health care direct practice and worthy of brief review for two reasons. First, they are components of evidence-based interventions, and, second, they foster the consumer's achieving new positive experiences early in the intervention process.

These techniques are normalizing; reframing; role-playing; and homework assignments. Briefly, normalizing refers to the practitioner acknowledging that consumer and family reactions to the stress or negative responses to the illness situation are common, and experienced by many consumers; normalizing itself may reduce stress (Corwin, 2002). Reframing involves the practitioner transposing—relabeling—the negative attribution(s) made by a consumer about, for instance, a diagnosis or a planned medical intervention, with a positive interpretation that fits the facts of the situation (Gambrill, 1997). Role-playing involves allowing the consumer to practice, with the social worker as coach, various alternative ways of responding to a situation (Corwin, 2002). Role-playing allows the consumer to try out, and then process with the worker, the pros and cons of various ways of approaching the issues. Homework assignments are tasks the client completes between sessions. Homework is a component of several brief intervention models, such as cognitive-behavioral interventions, because it extends the accomplishments of a session beyond the limits of that session into the everyday life of the client. In time-limited work such as in ambulatory health care settings, this attribute of homework tasks is particularly useful. The social worker and the consumer collaboratively develop an assignment, ideally by the end of the first session. Gambrill (1997) identified criteria for homework assignments, including

- empirical evidence suggests that completion of the assignment leads to desired outcomes;
- consumers can accomplish the assignment;
- barriers, and ways to overcome them, are specified;
- needed resources are supplied.

Homework prompts consumers to practice new solutions or coping strategies, and potentially enhance their sense of efficacy in managing their health condition. Incorporating self-monitoring and recording results in homework tasks, such as increased knowledge of their health condition and adherence to medication regimens or lifestyle changes, can substantiate progress, identify areas needing continuing intervention, and provide data for evaluation of outcomes. The burgeoning availability on the Internet of educational information designed specifically for health consumers, often with interactive components, is one resource for homework assignments (see Appendix B on Web site summaries).

There are three specific evidence-based and time-limited interventions appropriate for ambulatory social work practice: disease management; cognitive-behavioral treatment (CBT); and complementary/alternative medicine (CAM) interventions. Crisis intervention is, by definition, time limited and appropriate in ambulatory health care, though somewhat less rigorously evaluated for efficacy in ambulatory health care settings. Thus, the following discussion details these interventions and the role of social work in each in direct practice with individual consumers and their families and small groups.

Disease Management

The disease management models build on population-based medical guidelines and clinical outcome research, and CBT. Diseases appropriate for this intervention are those for which the most research knowledge is available (Hunter & Fairfield, 1997). Evaluation of disease management models for specific chronic and high-cost illnesses (e.g., diabetes, asthma, arthritis), which affect large numbers of consumers, documents improved health outcomes, cost efficiencies, and positive patient satisfaction (e.g., Claiborne, & Massaro, 2000; Ligon, 1998; Steinman, Steinman, & Steinman, 2003; Tinkelman & Schwartz, 2004).

Disease management is an integrated and client-centered, evidence-based intervention including medical, psychological, and psychosocial care, implemented across acute and less than acute episodes of illnesses through the involvement of all professionals. The consumer and providers coshare responsibility for management of the disease and for evaluating progress and outcomes (Claiborne & Vandenburgh, 2001; Hunter & Fairfield, 1997). The overall goals of disease management are

- reduction of the number and intensity of episodes of an illness and comorbid conditions;
- increased inpatient self-care capacities.

Disease management guidelines specify evidence-based psychosocial interventions, such as cognitive-behavioral interventions, and require the collection of objective medical and psychosocial data to evaluate both process and outcomes ideally via standardized scales and instruments. In contrast to behavioral health, which tends to focus on at-risk behaviors, such as unprotected sex and smoking, disease management presumes a relationship between psychosocial and person-in-environment factors, health-related behaviors, health outcomes, and quality of life.

The first premise of a disease management intervention is that the consumer and all providers are comprehensively knowledgeable about the patient's disease; the providers are responsible for establishing an effective support system and resources for individual consumers, and monitoring the results of interventions to ensure improvement. In disease management interventions, social work expertise in the relationship of psychosocial issues and health conditions can enhance the plan of care and its implementation and is therefore valuable to the team (Claiborne & Vandenburgh, 2001). Given the available evidence of effectiveness, it is heartening to the profession that disease management is clearly a biopsychosocial approach. One social work role in disease management is educating the consumers about their condition, medical information and care that might otherwise be presented only in complex medical terms, or, because of the time constraints imposed on physicians by managed care, without adequate time for consumers' questions, to facilitate self-management. Teaching consumers self-management skills involves specific steps:

- providing sufficient information geared to the consumers' cognitive ability to understand;
- developing activities (e.g., homework assignments) targeted at management of the symptoms of health conditions and concomitant feelings.

Getting information for educating clients is now easier due to the vast amount of health and health care information available on the Internet. Practitioners are strongly encouraged to evaluate the Web sites they refer consumers to because some, but only some, offer evidenced-based information and are amenable to layperson use (see Web site summaries in Appendix B).

Cultural Responsiveness in Disease Management

Remember that cultural background is dynamic and fluid, rather than a set of categorical determinations. Thus, attention to cultural responsiveness in disease management can improve the likelihood of clients' participation and adherence to interventions. Disease management is a linear model based on the biomedical model (i.e., identify problem, identify evidence-based intervention, measure outcomes). A consumer whose culturally related social rules or values favor non-direct communication, or whose spiritual orientation affirms universal body-mind-spirit harmony, or whose health beliefs are personalistic, rather than biomedical, may understandably be less than fully participatory. The social worker might normalize such hesitancies or reframe the seeming singular focus of disease management interventions on a physical condition to combinations of body, mind, and spirit.

Just as important to positive consumer outcomes in cross-cultural situations is the role of the social worker on the disease management team. Medical education does not often include cultural or psychosocial issues or content (e.g., Flores, 2000). This absence in training may limit physicians' detection of patients' cultural as well as psychosocial issues (DeCoster & Egan, 2001; Lesser, 2000; Simonian & Tarnowski, 2001). The social worker can educate the disease management interdisciplinary team about the cultural aspects and psychosocial problems of the consumer that can impinge on the health and quality of life outcomes, and that might deter the consumer's effective participation in care. Social work expertise in these areas helps the interdisciplinary team link medical clinical information and the consumer's psychosocial capacities and stressors and cultural background.

Practitioners' exploration of the role of values, health beliefs, and cultural background in relation to management of the disease can promote consumer participation with providers in the care plan. Problem-solving strategies can assist clients with becoming more skilled in self-care and capable in making health care decisions; teaching, coaching, role-playing, and teaching stress management skills can promote consumer participation and increase coping capacities.

In summary, disease management is an evidence-based, interdisciplinary intervention protocol in community-based health care for several major health conditions. Social workers' role capitalizes on expertise in the relationships of psychosocial and cultural factors, and health and illness. The monitoring and outcome evaluation components of disease management meet managed care requirements and supply practitioners with evidence to verify the effectiveness of their interventions.

Cognitive-Behavioral Interventions

Corwin (2002) notes that CBT facilitates establishing early rapport because it makes early positive change for the consumer possible. Because of this attribute and confirmation of efficacy, cognitive-behavioral interventions are particularly favored by managed care (Comer, 2004; Dziegielewski & Holliman, 2001). While an exhaustive discussion of CBT is outside the scope of this text, the following discussion presents an overview and the techniques inherent in the model applied to ambulatory health care consumer situations.

CBT is a structured approach directed toward the consumers learning that their unfounded schemas contribute or produce their problems, changing these faulty cognitions, and, thus, resolving problematic behaviors. CBT centers on changing a consumer's cognitions through systematically altering automatic thoughts and unfounded (i.e., irrational) beliefs/belief systems and ideas (Beck, 1995). CBT uses specific techniques, including role-playing, coaching, and homework assignments. While the client is a full participant, the practitioner actively leads and coaches the consumer. First steps include assisting the consumer in

- understanding and accepting the linkages between his or her thoughts and problems;
- committing to participate in changing those cognitions.

Examples, given by the social worker, that demonstrate the links between thoughts and behaviors are particularly useful. As a client realizes how irrational schema lead to unwanted behaviors, receptivity to changing these cognitions increases.

Remember Mrs. Thompson? Her client story and concerns are appropriate for cognitive-behavioral intervention. The second step is a detailed exploration of the beliefs, automatic thoughts, and self-statements (i.e., self-talk) concerning the identified problematic behavior or situation. Exploring Mrs. Thompson's cognitions (i.e., self-talk) about her medical problems and recommended lifestyle changes reveals the following beliefs:

- Physical problems, such as hypertension and high cholesterol, are "just genetic" and unalterable.
- Physical activity and reducing fat content in her diet cannot affect hypertension or high cholesterol anyway.

After exploration identifies automatic cognitions and schema that are barriers to achieving positive health outcomes, the practitioner then challenges Mrs. Thompson's automatic thoughts and unfounded beliefs concerning hypertension and high cholesterol, jogging and diet, and systematically suggests new—experience changing—more well-founded and rational beliefs. The social worker might ask, for example, "Mrs. Thompson, how did you come to concluding that health problems like yours are genetic and unalterable?" and asking for evidence of the validity of that conclusion. Further exploration could reveal that Mrs. Thompson also believes that

- she is incapable of achieving what she desires;
- she will just fail in any endeavor;
- God is in charge of her health.

Such negative self-statements often cluster with irrational health-related beliefs. In the process of further exploration, the clinician identifies factors that might interfere with change. Perhaps Mrs. Thompson's children share her beliefs about health. If so, the plan might be adjusted to include the daughters and/or assist Mrs. Thompson in effectively incorporating them in homework assignments. Next, the worker and Mrs. Thompson discuss potential new cognitions and identify the ones that can be successful and those that might not. Through reflective listening, the practitioner can model responses to these alternatives, coach Mrs. Thompson in implementing new cognitions, and lead her in discussing her feelings about implementing the new schema, while reinforcing success and identifying areas for improvement.

In brief, as the client becomes comfortable with connections between cognitions and lack of success in changing physical activity and diet, he or she is ready to monitor his or her thoughts outside the presence of the social worker. Practicing self-monitoring with the worker in a session is empowering and reinforces the process, as does the client keeping daily logs. Daily logs record

- thoughts/cognitions;
- associated feelings;
- success with new cognitions.

The log is valuable for the client because it helps him or her focus on the change, and for the clinician because logs identify progress and needed next steps.

Of course, it is best practice to evaluate the appropriateness of CBT with culturally diverse consumers (Comer, Kramer, & Nash, 2000). Clients from cultures that, for example, believe illness is caused by mind-body imbalances, or endorse less active or less cognitive methods, may be unlikely candidates for CBT. CBT might be inappropriate for clients who see the premises of CBT as flawed, whereas those who are more assimilated to the cause-effect links of Western medicine, or to using ethnocultural and Western health interventions in parallel care, may be more acceptant.

To sum up, a large body of research evidences the effectiveness of CBT. Cognitive-behavioral intervention is time-limited, focused, and elegantly structured intervention with multiple techniques for changing a variety of problematic behaviors making it very useful in ambulatory health care practice. CBT is identified as a best practice in disease management models, and is endorsed by managed care systems and in biomedical health care.

Crisis Intervention

Crisis reactions can occur in community health care given the possibility of a consumer receiving a life-altering diagnosis or needing a serious medical intervention. The following discussion provides an overview of the intervention.

In general, three types of events can prompt a crisis. A crisis may result from a threat associated with an anticipated loss (e.g., the possibility of a life-changing or terminal illness). Second, a crisis may stem from the possibility of a negative outcome (e.g., surgery or treatment to resolve a life-changing illness). Third, an overwhelming loss related to an event that has already occurred (e.g., amputation) can result in a crisis reaction. The purpose of crisis intervention is to restore the consumer's ability to function. Crisis intervention has several basic principles (Corwin, 2002; Hepworth, Rooney, & Larsen, 2002). These principles are

- reactions to a health care crisis are normative;
- the strengths perspective suggests that a consumer's usual coping capacity(ies) can be elicited to cope with the present health care crisis;
- the consumer can make good use of short-term interventions;
- the crisis is an opportunity to learn new coping strategies.

The first phase of a crisis is increasing stress and tension, with accompanying shock and, perhaps, denial during which clients are likely to resort to their usual emergency coping strategies. If these strategies fail, stress and tension continue to rise, leading consumers to feel confused and overwhelmed. In the second phase, consumers may try other strategies, which may or may not help; if these attempts are not successful in coping with the crisis, stress levels and feeling overwhelmed and confused escalate—the third phase of crisis. A client's response is contextualized by previous experiences with crises and is related to culturally varying attributions about the situation. Clearly, the earlier in the process that crisis intervention occurs, the more likely is success.

In ambulatory health care, the focus of crisis intervention is on the consumer's medical condition prompting the crisis. As in other settings, in crisis intervention the worker is active and leads the consumer through the process. Establishing rapid rapport is essential. In brief, crisis intervention involves exploring the client's feelings, and then normalizing these reactions is the first step in reducing stress. Education about the medical condition or diagnosis and planned medical care/interventions can also reduce stress. The clinician then explores the consumer's usual coping strategies and support systems and builds upon them in collaboration with consumer and family, when the latter is available, to develop a plan of action. Assisting the consumer in establishing a positive alliance with health care providers helps assure effective relationships for the duration of the medical care that may be initiated by the health crisis.

In brief, crisis intervention is a structured intervention in community health care for consumers who receive serious medical diagnoses or recommendations for treatment that initially overwhelm them.

Crisis intervention can stabilize the consumers through identifying and helping them use their coping resources; practitioners access resources the clients may need to maintain that stability.

Complementary and Alternative Medical Interventions

Increasingly interventions outside traditional biomedicine are implemented independently, or alongside, mainstream allopathic interventions (National Center for Complementary and Alternative Medicine, 2004). In medicine these are referred to as complementary or alternative medicine (CAM). Complementary interventions are used in conjunction with biomedicine, while alternative techniques are used instead of biomedical interventions. CAM interventions and products "are not presently considered part of conventional medicine" (National Center for Complementary and Alternative Medicine, 2002). In this discussion, the use of CAM is in relation to specific interventions, rather than alternative systems of health care, such as homeopathic medicine. In general, the purpose of many CAM interventions is to alter a physical reaction/state or increase a person's ability to cope with stress or enhance overall wellness. Their use in social work in ambulatory health care reflects the emphasis on consumer participation in care and social work's commitment to cultural diversity, since it may reflect a consumer's cultural worldview or health belief sets better than allopathic medicine.

CAM intervention techniques include educational and behavioral techniques that, overall, foster relaxation, used in multiple sessions, either with individual or in small groups of consumers, with sessions on specific techniques and homework assignments. The practitioner's objective is to teach specific techniques so that clients can use them in self-directed practice. Interventions include techniques to decrease a physical response to stress, such as increased breathing and heart rate, and muscle tension. Evidence suggests that relaxation techniques, including meditation, yoga, and guided imagery, are effective in reducing stress, anxiety, and chronic pain (Finger & Arnold, 2002). These three specific interventions are discussed in the following paragraph.

The objective of meditation is to relax the body and calm the mind. Techniques include focusing passively on a sensation in specific parts of the body (e.g., warmth in the arms, coolness of the forehead), breathing, or heart rate. Yoga techniques achieve relaxation through movement. Guided imagery often utilizes other relaxation techniques, such as focusing, and may be used for a specific condition, such as asthma or headaches, or more generally to allow a consumer to understand and reduce the impact of the stresses being experienced. Guided imagery is effective in reducing the severity and frequency of chronic tension headaches (Mannix, Chandurkar, Rybicki, Tusek, & Solomon, 1999) and cancer symptoms (Wallace, 1997).

Biofeedback can be incorporated in relaxation interventions. Biofeedback involves the client learning to monitor and regulate physical responses to stress, such as muscle tension, skin temperature, sweating, pulse or breathing rates, with mechanical instruments (e.g., blood pressure cuffs, heart monitors). Findings suggest that biofeedback is effective in reducing headaches, blood pressure, and pain in fibromyalgia (Finger & Arnold, 2002).

In sum, the utility of CAM interventions for social workers in community-based health settings is that they are not only evidence-based but also

- congruent with social work principles of empowerment and self-determination;
- flexible and can be adapted to the specific needs of individual consumers.

Social workers can learn each of the techniques discussed previously. The appropriateness of their use in health care practice with diverse consumers, whose cultural backgrounds endorse a body-mind-spirit connection, is evident (also see Appendix B on Web site summaries).

Using Advanced Health Technology with Individual Consumers/Families

Advances in health-related technology, including computer technology, are gaining increased use in individual/family ambulatory care to increase access to health information, services, and resources.

As one illustration of the psychosocial benefit of advanced technologies, computer technology in assistive devices now allows persons with Lou Gehrig's disease (i.e., amyotrophic lateral sclerosis, or ALS) to record statements in their own voice before the disease destroys their ability to speak (Amyotrophic Lateral Sclerosis Association, 2004). The technology, allowing the consumer to continue communicating with family throughout this devastating terminal illness regardless of disease stage, is dramatic and beneficial. Other devices make lifelong medical treatments, such as blood sugar monitoring and insulin injections, less complex and uncomfortable.

Examples of using telehealth technology to deliver services appeared in a previous chapter (Chapter 4). Also of note is the array of disease-specific Web sites that include information, online support groups, and economical access to medical resources. These Web sites are resources for practitioners in direct practice to help consumers gain information and support resources. The challenge for practitioners is to incorporate current knowledge of technological resources for clients and to critically analyze the utility and appropriateness of these technologies in direct practice with consumers. The Web site summaries in Appendix B present many relevant Web sites that were critically analyzed for their appropriateness and utility to direct practice.

Small Group Work in Community Health Care

Time-limited small group work is gaining favor with managed care because it serves a number of consumers simultaneously, and there is evidence substantiating that it is as effective as interventions with individuals. Group interventions have a long history of acceptance in mental health practice, and are part of social work's standard armamentarium. Empirical evidence of the effectiveness of small group interventions in health care practice is growing. As illustrations, recent research findings indicate that small group interventions are effective in

- reducing the prevalence of teen pregnancy (Franklin & Corcoran, 2000);
- increasing the problem-solving ability of teen mothers and parents (Harris & Franklin, 2003);
- improving coping and decreasing stress in HIV+ patients (Cruess et al., 2002);

- reducing negative health and psychosocial outcomes for persons with sickle cell disease (Comer, 2004);
- reducing emergency room use and hospitalizations (Scott et al., 2004).

Increasing evidence also supports the efficacy of small group interventions with consumers of diverse cultural backgrounds (Comer, 2004; Comer, Kramer, & Nash, 2000; Leon & Dziegielewski, 2000).

Time-limited small group interventions are appropriate in community-based health care social work because this modality can be effective in meeting several areas of consumer needs, such as increasing knowledge of medical conditions and care, reducing the stress of a chronic illness, improving coping capacities, and changing behaviors, beliefs, and attitudes related to health conditions and diseases.

Planning Steps for Initiating Small Groups

Planning steps for initiating small groups are pivotal in effectiveness. Consideration of "who" is generating the idea of forming the group is a first step; the idea may come from social workers, colleagues, management, or clients. Several questions for planning small group interventions are pertinent in ambulatory health care settings (Gambrill, 1997; Tolson, Reid, & Garvin, 2002):

- Is official authorization needed or useful?
- What type of group intervention(s) will be used? When will the group meet? How often? For how long?
- For which, and how many, consumers? Is the group to be open or closed?
- What resources (e.g., space, leader(s), materials) are needed?

In some instances an official authorization for implementing a group from agency management, clinical directors, and so on, is necessary and useful to acquiring resources. Coordinating the time schedule of planned group meetings is particularly important in primary care and clinic settings so that patient appointments and group schedules are compatible, and group meeting space is available.

The type of group (i.e., psychoeducational, social support, intervention or a combination) and the intervention modality(ies) (e.g., cognitive-behavioral, disease management, education, or a combination) must be in line with needs of members, the purpose, and the desired outcome(s) of the group (Comer, 2004). Small group interventions can incorporate disease management interventions (e.g., education, monitoring, cognitive-behavioral).

The overall desired outcomes for groups in ambulatory care help determine the type of group. For instance, the purpose of psychoeducational groups is that members gain knowledge and coping skills related to a health problem or need. The goal of social support groups is to increase the support system of members and thereby enhance coping capacities by providing members with the opportunity to share and hear the experiences of others who have the same disease and to find that one's personal reactions and concerns are typical (i.e., normalizing). The purpose of intervention groups is a change or changes in individual members (e.g., lifestyle behaviors, health cognitions, coping capacities).

Given the desired outcome, type of group, and type of intervention, determining the appropriate group size, the length and number of group sessions, and whether the group is to be closed (i.e., no new members after the initial meeting) or open (i.e., new members may join at any point) logically follows. The size of a group is generally determined by its purpose; purely educational and support groups tend to be somewhat larger (e.g., ≥ 10 members) than intervention groups (e.g., ≤ 10 members). Space and staff resources and/or the target group of consumers may influence the length and/or number of group sessions. In the case of an intervention group, the length and number of sessions can be governed by the time required for the effective implementation. In general, a closed group structure is more appropriate to time-limited ambulatory health care because group cohesion occurs more quickly.

A concrete consideration is to determine what resources are needed to implement the group. These include space for meetings, skilled leader(s), access to the building if a group is to meet after normal hours of operation, and possibly care for members' children. All requirements as discussed previously (e.g., consents) are established before the initial group meeting. Group norms (i.e., accepted rules and behaviors), such as confidentiality in the group and expectations for attendance, may be preset, or an objective of the initial group meeting.

Recruiting and screening of members for a group is basic to planning groups. Recruiting and screening potential members should assure that a potential member is

- capable of benefiting from the group;
- appropriate to a group intervention given the current needs;
- comparable to other members in health condition or problems.

For instance, a small group may not be best practice for a consumer/family who has just received a diagnosis of a life-changing illness, because their capability to benefit and current needs are not appropriate to being in a group at this time. In time-limited health care practice, the homogeneity of group members, whether they are consumers, family members, or caregivers, is important to facilitate timely group cohesion.

A comprehensive discussion of the specific steps in implementing the first session of a group is beyond the scope of this book. In brief, however, the initial meeting of the group has several objectives:

- helping members get to know one another;
- discussing the common ground of the health condition or concern;
- discussing and agreeing on the goals and rules of the group.

These activities begin the process of group formation and cohesion—the degree to which members feel part of a common group experience—and prompt members to share and assist other members. Discussing and commitment to group norms, with particular attention to confidentiality and attendance norms, is important in a first session.

In sum, groups in community health are planned and structured. As an example of a time-limited group in ambulatory health care practice, Comer (2004) describes planning of a support and educational group intervention for persons with sickle cell anemia. An interdisciplinary team, including social workers, in a comprehensive medical setting planned the structure, goal, and interventions with the aim of enhancing coping and increasing knowledge about sickle cell of group members. Potential members were patients with sickle cell between the ages of eighteen and sixty; ten of the twenty-five patients screened were found appropriate for the closed group. Initial sessions attended to shared issues and expectations for attendance and confidentiality. Cognitive-behavioral interventions occurred throughout the eight weekly ninety-minute sessions, including topics on knowledge of the disease, feelings of depression associated with sickle cell, and the linkages between negative thought patterns and depression.

In brief, time-limited small groups can incorporate cognitive-behavioral, psychoeducation, and disease management interventions. Planning for small groups is essential, including defining the size, type, and duration of the group, and the interventions. Small group work in community-based health care—like practice with individuals—is focused and time limited.

Telecommunication Technology in Small Group Work

The use of telecommunication technology for group work is expanding. Telecommunication can deliver prevention, social support, and psychoeducational group interventions. Evaluation studies of small groups offered via telecommunication technology substantiate their efficacy (e.g., Heckman et al., 1999; Roffman et al., 1997). By the mid-1990s, social work began delivering group services via telephone conferencing to meet the needs of consumers geographically distant from providers (Galinsky, Schopler, & Abell, 1997; McCarty & Clancy, 2002). McCarty and Clancy (2002) note several issues to keep in mind when considering providing direct interventions via telehealth technologies, including assurance that the technology is sufficiently stable to guarantee consistent availability and quality, access is available for any consumer wishing to be a recipient, and privacy and confidentiality are secure.

Applying the Logic Modeling Technique with Mrs. Thompson

As a summary application of the interventions discussed, the following applies logic modeling to a consumer scenario. The logic model technique was applied earlier in this chapter to the consumer scenario of Mrs. Thompson in describing the problem statement of the current situation, identifying the list of problems to be resolved, and related expected objectives of interventions. Given the assessment noted previously, the problem list, and objectives, and presentation of cognitive-behavioral interventions with Mrs. Thompson, the methods section of the model might also include a psychoeducational support group and possibly biofeedback techniques to control blood pressure.

ETHICAL DILEMMAS IN DIRECT PRACTICE

As indicated in an earlier chapter, an ethical conflict occurs when a practitioner finds that two or more ethical principles apply to a situation, and that adhering to either results in a negative outcome. There is nothing pleasant about experiencing an ethical dilemma. Moreover, there is nothing simple about analyzing an ethical dilemma. Several recommendations for analyzing and resolving ethical dilemmas are available in the literature (e.g., Congress, 2004; Dodd & Jansson, 2004; Lowenberg, Dolgoff, & Harrington, 2000). Social workers' first ethical obligation is identifying when an ethical dilemma happens, or can potentially occur, their related personal values, and the values of the setting (Congress, 2000). Consistent recommendations for analyzing and resolving ethical dilemmas include

- identifying competing principles via the NASW *Code of Ethics;*
- comparing the positive and negative outcomes of each competing principle;
- prioritizing outcomes based on primary obligations to client well-being and subsidiary obligations to confidentiality, employer financial well-being, and so on;
- consulting with supervisors and others.

Lowenberg and coauthors (2000) place the highest ethical obligation on protecting and sustaining life, and the lowest on truthfulness. They note that biomedical (i.e., physicians and nurses) ethics also place the highest professional value on protection and preservation of life. For instance, social workers may be challenged when the results of a biomedical intervention that can sustain a consumer's life can also have potentially negative psychosocial effects, such as those discussed in a previous chapter concerning genetic predisposition testing. While all authors on ethical dilemmas recommend consultation with supervisors, in community-based health care settings, one's supervisor may be of a profession other than social work; being part of a professional network of social workers is, therefore, particularly important.

Ethical dilemmas in managed health care settings often involve client confidentiality and self-determination. In aggregate, transparency with consumers about the limits of confidentiality (Millstein, 2000) and the transfer of consumer information is necessary (National Association of Social Workers, 2001). Dodd and Jansson (2004) note that social workers are obliged to support client self-determination and urge practitioners to advocate and to help health care consumers bring their issues and questions directly to providers; the latter is empowering and addresses the profession's ethical commitment to consumer self-determination. Technological advances raise ethical considerations, as well. For example, as noted previously, security and confidentiality must be assured when services are delivered via telehealth technologies. The availability of genetic testing raises several potential ethical dilemmas including third party access to test results: What are insurers or managed care systems likely to do with the information?

However, some dilemmas are not *ethical* dilemmas but *practice* dilemmas. The differences between these are at times few. For instance, consumers who do not follow through with homework assignments, are consistently late for appointments, or divulge new information only at the end of a session do not present ethical dilemmas. While these instances are troubling to practitioners, they do not present ethical dilemmas—they present practice dilemmas.

In contrast, health consumers telling the practitioners that the physician is demeaning or does not listen concerning their beliefs about their condition does constitute ethical conflicts about the confidentiality and obligations to colleagues and consumers. Following the process detailed previously, the worker first identifies the principles involved, and compares the results. On the one hand, speaking with the physician can abridge client confidentiality; on the other hand, suggesting that the doctor's behavior is acceptable demeans the consumer and his or her right to self-determination. Ethical obligations to protect confidentiality and self-determination might be addressed by helping the consumer develop strategies to change his or her interactions with providers. The ethical dilemma could extend further were the physician to speak to the social worker describing the same client as "difficult." The practitioner now faces abridging consumer confidentiality and assuring client well-being, or being dishonest with colleagues. Resolutions in the latter situation could include

- suggesting strategies to the physician for improving interactions with clients;
- volunteering to do an in-service on working with patients perceived as difficult.

It is relevant to note that astute practitioners routinely discuss their role overall and ethical obligations at the beginning of work with consumers, and reinforce these with interdisciplinary colleagues as a matter of course, without reference to specific clients.

INTERDISCIPLINARY HEALTH CARE TEAMS

Managed care systems endorse the development and implementation of comprehensive care plans by interdisciplinary teams, rather than by single providers. Thus, it behooves social workers in community-based health care settings to be highly knowledgeable and skilled in effective interdisciplinary teamwork. In the present discussion, teamwork relates to interdisciplinary collaboration within a setting (i.e., intra-agency).

Most of the research on social work in interdisciplinary teams involves doctor– or nurse–social work collaboration. Of note, though reflecting specifically on collaboration with psychiatrists for medication referrals, Bentley and coauthors identify the importance of social workers understanding dissonance in professional perspectives, language, and "assumptions about human behaviors" (Bentley, Walsh, & Farmer, 2005, p. 62) as have others (Abramson & Mizrahi, 2003). A study of collaboration in community-based primary care found that collaborating social workers became the "eyes and ears" of physicians (Netting & Williams, 2000, p. 237). These authors suggest that direct practice with consumers with complex psychosocial needs may overwhelm physicians, whereas social workers see these patients more positively as just challenges. Techniques to demonstrating expertise in these instances are

- actively making collaborative connections with primary care physicians;
- linking consumers' psychosocial and health issues with the priority to demonstrate positive health outcomes to managed care systems and third party payers.

One strength that social work brings to ambulatory health care is the knowledge that health, illness, and psychosocial and cultural factors interact. Practitioners demonstrate expertise and professionalism, especially with medically trained colleagues, when they link psychosocial and cultural issues with consumer participation and compliance to medical care with psychosocial issues and demonstrate how psychosocial content can enhance achieving health outcomes.

Consultations are an opportunity to show social work expertise in resolving barriers to the team's successful intervention that psychosocial issues of the client and/or family could create. Moreover, consistency over time in consultation and education with interdisciplinary colleagues is pivotal in establishing lasting functional collaboration (Cameron & Mauksch, 2002). Consultations and education with team members might concern

- a specific consumer and his or her psychosocial needs that impact successful compliance with care and health outcomes;
- use of empirically validated screening tools and evaluating outcomes;
- psychosocial impact of issues pertaining to a group or population of consumers, such as
  1. typical emotional reactions to the initial diagnosis of an acute or chronic illness;
  2. the emotional, psychosocial impact of a diagnosis or chronic illness at different points in the lifespan, such as
     a. diagnosis of multiple sclerosis during early adulthood;
     b. families managing the asthma of their children as they enter adolescence.

Practitioners who demonstrate effectiveness in reducing duplication of services, no-show rates, and preventing failures in health outcome achievement are valued as collaborators. Offering education on evidence-based screening and assessment instruments helps establish professional credibility because medically trained colleagues value science-based knowledge. Social workers can strengthen their role as collaborators by convening, and actively facilitating the process of, team meetings. Techniques that foster effectiveness in small groups, such as reflective listening and redirecting to the topic at hand, can be effective in team meetings since teams are essentially a small group.

Barriers to Effective Teamwork

Interdisciplinary team members bring varying professional values and perspectives of consumers' needs. For instance, medical colleagues may see the interventions needed with a newly diagnosed diabetic as learning how to control glucose levels and/or how to inject insulin, whereas the social worker may see the need as feeling competent in coping with the stress of having diabetes and hopeful about self-care. Each is true, and they interlink. In illustration, Exhibit 5.1 very briefly depicts varying professional interventions with the parents of a nine-year-old child whose asthma attacks are increasing in severity and frequency.

The exhibit shows how a professional lens shapes the identification of how to resolve consumer health issues and problems. All disciplines bring their profession's knowledge, skills, language, jargon, and differing ways of solving problems to the team, while having limited understanding of these same areas of the other disciplines. Open communication can be disrupted when the team does not have a language that can be mutually understood with which to describe

---

EXHIBIT 5.1. An example of professional differences for a patient and family's intervention needs.

Medical and/or nursing	Social work assessment
• monitor child for early symptoms of an attack • learn how to correctly implement medication • know side effects of medication	• increase capacities for coping with the stress of parenting a chronically ill child • grieve the loss of having "a completely healthy child" • collaborate with the child's teacher

consumers, and one another. Social workers can help with this translation in teamwork and with consumers.

Physicians and nurses trained in the Western medical model truly see consumers as their responsibility—understandably given their respective professional codes and the regulations of managed care. Social workers become valued colleagues when our expanded view of consumers—as embedded in social, familial, cultural, and ecological systems—is linked to positive health outcomes. Confusion about the social work role and expertise in health care can result in "turf protection" by colleagues of other disciplines. However, such conflicts can be prevented and overcome through demonstrating mutual respect, commitment, and credibility, and acknowledging the benefits of having multiple knowledge bases and areas of expertise to the team (Abramson & Mizrahi, 2003; Congress, 2000).

COORDINATING AN INDIVIDUAL CONSUMER'S CARE

The paradigm shift in health care that emphasizes effectiveness, prevention, and wellness prompts attention to coordinating care in community health. Care coordination, a more consumer-centered term than case coordination—the latter connoting a crate holding some type of commodity—is a process of organizing existing services, augmenting services, and advocating for clients (Chernesky & Grube, 2000; Corwin, 2002). Care coordination is central to implementing continuous and efficient care, especially for consumer populations with chronic illnesses, multiple psychosocial needs, and/or limited resources.

Unhappily, care coordination is a term used widely, but inconsistently and ambiguously; though most assume they are consistent and clear. Just as mistakenly, some presume that care coordination assures an equitable distribution of resources/services and cost savings. Unfortunately, the quality of care coordination can suffer from these presumptions and definitional ambiguity, as well as from role, power, and authority conflicts. Definitional ambiguity can confound a plan for a continuum of health care when agencies to which a consumer is referred function with varying understandings of what coordination entails, and what their respective roles and responsibilities are. Actually coordinating care—preventing gaps and redundancies in care—can conflict with the territoriality, market share, or revenue streams that one or more agencies in the coordination plan hold dear. Though myths may persist and potential conflicts exist, care coordination does have several potential strengths:

- resolving gaps in service by locating needed resources;
- adaptability to transient change(s) in service systems and/or consumer needs;
- accountability;
- enhanced effectiveness and efficiency in service provision.

Care coordination within a health care setting by a single social worker for the consumers and their families with whom the worker directly practices is the basic and most simple model of care coordination (i.e., client-by-client coordination). Best practice suggests that direct feedback loops from consumers and from referred-to resources to the originating social worker are essential in maintaining a continuity of care, in meeting the profession's ethical obligation to consumer's well-being, and in avoiding client abandonment (National Association of Social Workers, 2001). However, feedback loops are not necessarily in place. Figure 5.3 shows care coordination by a single social worker within a health care setting; solid lines show referrals to resources and dotted lines indicate desirable feedback loops.

A variant of the care coordination depicted in Figure 5.3 (i.e., one social worker making referrals for his or her own clients one by one)

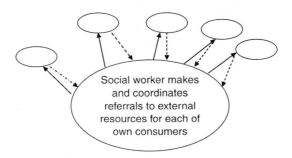

FIGURE 5.3. Client-by-client care coordination by a single practitioner in a health care setting.

is care coordination by one employee of an organization for all consumers of that setting. While this model may be appealing in terms of a unitary job position, and possibly agency billing for care coordination, it may be no more likely to have feedback loops to ensure quality and effective continuity of care.

Ethical Considerations in Interdisciplinary Care Coordination

Ethical considerations in coordinating care in interdisciplinary ambulatory health care settings for individual consumers involve the potential for conflicts between client and agency priorities and, thus, conflicting practitioner loyalties to the well-being of clients and to the employing agency. For instance, a client's needs for continuing and quality care and limitations in coverage of the worker's agency may conflict. In this regard, the *Code of Ethics* (NASW, 2001) advises workers to be knowledgeable about organizational policies on, and to clearly inform clients about, coverage and financial priorities. Also of relevance is the ethical obligation to avoid abandoning clients—to assure that clients they refer out of their practice will receive timely services of quality, or to continue service without coverage. This mandate requires workers to have up-to-date knowledge of the resources to which they refer, and to monitor—even without feedback loops formally in place—the clients after referral. The social worker may encounter ethical obligations to consumer well-being and continuity of care when interdisciplinary colleagues, having a differing viewpoint on consumer needs, may not see the priority of assuring quality and timely referrals.

Care coordination can result in practice, as well as ethical, dilemmas when the multiple agencies providing services to a consumer behave as independent "captains" of the client's care. On the one hand, territoriality may confound coordination, while, on the other, it conflicts with the professional obligation to consumer welfare.

In summary, care coordination in direct practice is an integrated intervention to organize, augment, and monitor a system of care for clients, ideally with built-in feedback loops. Ethical considerations arise when a practitioner's organization has financial priorities that conflict with client needs and/or when agencies referred to do not provide quality and timely services.

SUMMARY

In conclusion, the perspectives, concepts, and theories for practice in ambulatory care are

- strengths, ecological, and family systems perspectives;
- cognitive-behavioral and stress and coping theories.

Discussions explicated culturally responsive engagement and assessment concepts and techniques. Specific evidenced-based interventions for direct practice included disease management, cognitive-behavioral, complementary and alternative health, and small groups.

The basis and phases of crisis intervention and care coordination with individual consumers and their families were also explored. In addition, the chapter detailed logic modeling and applied logic modeling to consumer stories from assessment through intervention. Ethical considerations were highlighted throughout the chapter. In brief, ethical considerations in ambulatory health care direct practice center on client confidentiality, self-determination, and well-being versus agency priorities and varying professional viewpoints of consumers' needs for services.

DISCUSSION QUESTIONS AND ACTIVITIES FOR INDIVIDUALS AND SMALL GROUPS

1. Using the assessment and logic model presented in this chapter for Mrs. Thompson as a beginning, revise the assessment concepts and theories process and the logic model were the consumer to be the following:
   a. an African-American male;
   b. a recent woman immigrant from the Middle East with limited English;
   c. Latino male who is a member of a sexual minority;
   d. an employed white male without any health care coverage.
2. What are the ethical considerations in relation to each of the previous four consumers? Which consumers would be most difficult for you as the practitioner given your personal cultural background and values?

GLOSSARY

advocacy: Practice activities in direct practice targeted at educating, informing, or representing the needs and wishes of consumers with colleagues, agency management, or third-party payers.

alliance: A relationship between the practitioner and the consumer and consumer's family.

alternative/complementary health care: Alternative health care interventions, practices, and products not accepted by biomedicine; complementary approaches are generally accepted because of empirical evidence and used in conjunction with biomedicine.

assessment: The process of collecting consumer information/data and applying biopsychosocial concepts to understand the data/information and the consumer's situation and problems.

care coordination: The process of organizing existing services, seeking additional services, and advocating for clients.

cognitive-behavioral intervention: An intervention that incorporates behaviorism, social learning, and cognition theories and concepts in structured, planned short-term interventions.

collaboration: Multiple professionals working together to develop and implement a plan of care; may be interdisciplinary (an integrated endeavor) or multidisciplinary (a parallel endeavor without integration).

disease management: A client-centered, evidence-based model that includes medical, psychological, and psychosocial interventions that are integrated and implemented by interdisciplinary teams.

schema: A cognitive-behavioral term for patterns of thinking, cognitions, or beliefs.

Chapter 6

Practice on Behalf of Health Care Consumer Populations

- *What is practice on behalf of health care consumer populations?*
- *What are the relevant concepts for practice?*
- *What specific processes inform understanding for practice?*
- *What are the challenges to success in practice with multiple organizations and groups?*
- *What is "community health promotion and wellness"?*
- *How can social workers be effective leaders on behalf of consumers?*
- *What are the ethical dilemmas and value issues in practice on behalf of consumer populations?*

WHAT IS PRACTICE ON BEHALF OF HEALTH CARE CONSUMER POPULATIONS?

As noted previously, social work in ambulatory health care does not fit cleanly into either direct or indirect practice of knowledge and skills. Community-based health care practitioners are just as likely to work directly with clients as on behalf of larger groups or populations of health care consumers. Community-based health care practice reflects the suggestion that social work by definition involves change activities inclusive of micro and macro practice (Netting, Kettner, & McMurty, 2004).

Social Work Practice in Community-Based Health Care
© 2007 by The Haworth Press, Inc. All rights reserved.
doi:10.1300/5273_06

Practice on behalf of health care consumer populations or groups includes activities with and among organizations or agencies that provide services for clients with a particular health condition, or health risk factor(s), or in a particular geographic area, as well as with consumer and community groups. Practice on behalf of consumers is distinguished, therefore, from practice within an organization or agency where a social worker might develop an intervention for a group of clients of that agency. Thus, these activities in sum combine elements of organizational and community practice in planning and developing programs in the community for the benefit of a consumer population (e.g., Dunlop & Angell, 2001). As shaped to community-based health care practice, these include

- understanding communities, health care organizations, and agencies;
- assessing the needs of culturally diverse communities and health care consumer populations and health conditions;
- developing culturally responsive interorganizational and community collaborations, coalitions, and consortia;
- training and leading;
- evaluating programs.

Accordingly, this chapter discusses knowledge and approaches for planning and developing health programs and projects in community settings, particularly for at-risk consumer populations. It is beyond the intent of this chapter to explore the full extent of macro-administrative and community health care practice. Rather, the chapter consolidates the knowledge, concepts, practice approaches, and skills from several literature sources on social work administration and community practice as are relevant to social work practice in community-based practice on behalf of groups and populations of health consumers (Gibelman, 2003; Hardina, 2002; Netting, Kettner, & McMurty, 2004).

The chapter presents two particular strategies that are prevalent in health care practice on behalf of populations: collaborations and co-alitions/consortia. In addition, the chapter provides empirical examples of health care programs that reflect the concepts and employ the strategies presented to resolve fragmented health services and unmet consumer population needs. Relevant ethical considerations are included as appropriate. Evaluation of programs in ambulatory health care is a topic in Chapter 7 on evaluating practice and programs.

Clarification of some of the terms in the chapter will be helpful. The terms "consumer population(s)" and "consumer group(s)" are used interchangeably, as are the terms "interorganization" and "interagency" in reference to activities among and across systems and settings in the community. "Consumer group" and "consumer population" are terms that refer to a large number of persons who share health risk factors (e.g., predisposition to a disease, lack of health coverage), unmet needs (e.g., accessible primary care), and/or a geographical area (e.g., inner city, neighborhood).

CONCEPTS FOR PRACTICE: ORGANIZATIONS, COMMUNITIES, HEALTH CARE POPULATIONS, AND PROBLEMS

Practice on behalf of health consumer groups benefits from concepts for planning, assessment, and interventions. Ambulatory health care practice for consumer groups and populations most often involves work with and across multiple organizations and settings, and community groups. Therefore, understanding organizations, communities, as well as health care consumer populations and problems is requisite.

Organizations

Several basic concepts inform understanding organizations whether a practitioner's activities are in collaboratives, coalitions, or consortia. The organizations in this discussion are those that already serve the health care population or problem of interest, or that have a philosophical commitment or loyalty to either. Several characteristics and dynamics generic to human service organizations are pertinent to community-based health care practice on behalf of populations, including

- control;
- structure;

- decision making and authority;
- relationships;
- culture.

Organizational Control

Organizational control refers to the ways that power and influence are implemented within the organization (Netting, Kettner, & McMurty, 2004). The influence of an organization or an agency may extend beyond its boundaries to the community due to its long-term status or to the status of the organization's leader(s) in the community. Power and influence dynamics have particular implications when organizations commit to working with other organizations on behalf of consumers. For example, working together to resolve fragmented health care services for the working poor may challenge one or more organizations' routine control of their setting or staff. That is, joining with other organizations or agencies may mean giving over some control to the collective control of a multiorganizational group or team (Dunlop & Angell, 2001).

Organizational Structure

Organizational structure refers to the ways that roles and relationships are configured inside the setting (Gibelman, 2003). The structures of bureaucracies and corporations are clearly specified and are formally mandated by law or public policy. Agencies with hierarchical structures have clear lines of authority, communication, and roles, with a single or few persons in authority at the top. For example, health departments are hierarchical; clinics within health departments follow the hierarchical structure, with specified roles often determined by professional identification (e.g., nursing, medical, social work) or activity (e.g., community outreach).

In terms of financial structure, health care organizations may be public and nonprofit, such as health departments, or for-profit and proprietary. As discussed in an earlier chapter, health care organizations are increasingly proprietary. In comparison, community-based health care programs are often less hierarchical, and more often nonprofit.

Organizational Decision Making and Authority

Authority may be described as legitimate or charismatic. Legitimate authority derives from expertise and formal rules, whereas charismatic authority arises from personal attributes and history (Netting, Kettner, & McMurty, 2004). In general, decisions are of two types. In one type, decisions are unilateral, or centralized, and made by those in top authority; in the second type, decision making is decentralized, with decisions made less by top administrators and more by direct service providers, and/or by informal agreement among those directly involved. Gibelman (2003) suggests that informal decision making develops through psychosocial interactions inside an organization and determines how, and by whom, work activities occur.

Several recent authors identify the importance of consensual decision making by all involved, including consumers, in planning and implementing community-based health care initiatives for consumer groups (Arches, 2001; Auslander, Haire-Joshu, Houston, Williams, & Krebill, 2000; Bowie & Rocha, 2004; Hatchett & Duran, 2002; Thompson, Minkler, Bell, Rose, & Butler, 2003). In illustration, Hatchett and Duran (2002) link consensual decision making in a health prevention project by including "the voices and visions of persons previously excluded from decision making" (p. 44).

Relationships in Organizations

Relationships in an organizational context in ambulatory health care can relate to the status of individuals and organizations and the influence of managed care on agencies. For social workers in community-based health care practice on behalf of consumers, relationships can also be influenced by whether the settings are host settings (Gibelman, 2003).

Relationships evident in organizations, and in community-based practice on behalf of health consumers, may be personal, professional, or a combination of both. Personal relationships within organizations usually originate from shared work tasks or roles, and evolve, as trust grows, through frequent, often daily, interactions. These relationships may occur within the context of interorganizational activities, or predate them. Personal relationships can be strengths in practice on behalf of consumer groups when preexisting relationships are positive and the parties share similar perspectives on joint efforts and goals. Conversely, personal relationships can undermine achieving objectives if loyalty to the personal overrides commitment to a program, or interferes with effective planning. Professional relationships arise from identification with a specific discipline, or area of expertise (e.g., social work, nursing, health administration).

In any health care setting, there is often differential status attributed to one or more health care professions with the medical profession traditionally being ascribed the highest status. The identification by managed care of the physician as the accountable provider in health care settings reinforces that attribution. Potentially countering the status of physicians is the corollary endorsement of managed care for interdisciplinary care planning and services. The status attributed to one or another profession can interfere with interorganizational community health planning and development. Adding to the challenge of working with multiple organizations in practice on behalf of health care consumers, each with the characteristics discussed previously, is the likelihood that most of the organizations involved are likely to be host settings for social work.

Further, as noted in previous chapters, community-based health care practice is inherently interdisciplinary. Therefore, it is likely that social work practice on behalf of health consumer groups includes professionals within a single discipline, but whose roles vary—such as administrators, staff, or clinicians—and/or professionals from various disciplines who share similar roles—such as program managers. In either case, the commonality of a discipline or of a role can foster similar thinking that facilitates cohesion and efficient program planning and development, or it can be potentially divisive along disciplinary lines or roles.

By way of an illustration of disciplinary loyalties fostering divisions, Powell and colleagues (1999) describe the process of developing an interagency-university-consumer collaborative team innovation to meet the needs of children with severe emotional disturbances. They note the importance of strong relationships among members; solid collaborations must be "built on mutual respect . . . shared goals, a shared vision" (Powell et al., 1999, p. 46). They attribute strong personal and discipline-specific relationships, perspectives, and alliances to an ultimate split in the program. In sum, professional identities can create divisions or conflict as well as strengthen joint work. Therefore, practice on behalf of health care populations, as in direct practice, necessitates effective interdisciplinary skills and routinely educating colleagues about social work expertise, ethic, and value bases.

Professional perspectives might be demonstrated when an interdisciplinary and interorganizational planning group visits a faith-based clinic to assess the possibility of collaboration with the clinic in an interorganizational educational program for the population of adult diabetics in a community. So, let us imagine a situation in which we overhear the professionals in a discussion after such a visit:

> The administrator comments on the expansive amount of unused space which the project could utilize, while the social worker comments on the darkness of the waiting room, the glassed-in—with keyhole opening—receptionist cubicle, and that physicians were of one cultural group and gender, and consumers of others. The nurse and physician note the large number of nurses and size of the central station in the examination room area, and that exam rooms had curtains, but no doors, and the large number of clients. The discussion included observing some discomfort with the faith-related inscriptions.

A recent study of professional identity and perspective in interdisciplinary health care collaboration is illuminating. King and Ross (2003) studied relationships in a community-based interdisciplinary setting to discern how professional identity might enhance or deter the development of effective collaboration. The study was carried out in Britain, where the emphasis on interdisciplinary collaboration and planned care is as strong as in the United States. Recommendations to overcome barriers arising from professional identity are particularly salient to this discussion for their creativity and specificity. Specific strategies include to

- invest sufficient time in planning and training to
  1. clarify role ambiguities with team members and consumers;
  2. discuss and define roles and equitable workload of each profession;
  3. engender a flexible attitude about how tasks will occur;

- build on existing personal and work relationships among members of the team;
- ensure that work activities are colocated.

King and Ross (2003) offer creative "how to" strategies for resolving interprofessional identity issues. Some of the strategies include professionals shadowing each other at work during training to achieve a reality-based, rather than abstract, understanding of each other's roles and expertise, and including consumers throughout the process of planning and development.

Organizational Culture

Organizational culture—the patterns of behavior within an organization and in interactions of the organization with its external environment—develops from the shared experiences of its members in adaptation to both internal and external forces (Glisson, 2000). Organizational culture is similar to cultural background (explored in Chapter 3) in that it includes values and norms of behavior; it is an internal phenomenon of the organization relating to

- ways of accomplishing the agency's goals and objectives;
- patterns of informal relationships;
- perceptions of the purposes and outside relationships.

In summary, organizations have structures, authority, and decision-making patterns, and culture. As is true for individuals and groups, these dynamics interact and change over time through influences of the larger community and society. A conceptual framework for ambulatory health care practice on behalf of consumer groups, in addition to guiding understanding of organizations, includes knowledge of health consumer populations and problems.

Understanding the Community, Health Consumer Population, and Problems

Social work on behalf of health care consumer groups centers on two major problems for consumers: fragmented health service systems and unmet health needs. A process generic to effectively developing and planning community programs and projects guides planning to address these two major issues. The reader is reminded that a health consumer population may be a large number of persons with a specific health concern or medical condition, or who are at risk for a certain health condition, or who share a psychosocial characteristic, such as age or a geographic area, such as a school district. Organizations in this discussion are those involved or committed to the health care population or problem.

Understanding Communities

Understanding communities begins with an overview of their general functions from an ecological perspective. Communities are systems that provide social participation, socializing to the cultural norms and identity of their members, the production, distribution, and use of services and goods; community functions are interactive and not discrete entities (Hardina, 2002; Netting, Kettner, & McMurty, 2004). Applying the ecological systems perspective suggests that changes in one function, or constituent group, are likely to affect other functions and groups. In an environment of limited resources, it is true, more than ever, that communities must compete for all types of resources, including economic, social, and, of pertinence to this discussion, health care. The ripple effects of change within a community are germane to ambulatory health care social work because practice seeks community participation and change in the production and distribution of health services.

Communities have shared social values and norms of behavior, beliefs, and history, often related to the cultural background of constituents, that compositely contribute to a community identity. Netting and coauthors (2004) note that a community generally includes trusted social networks, and in place organizations that contribute to the stability and resilience of the community. Analyzing a community in relation to community-based health includes understanding several aspects of a community, including

- social and economic history;
- beliefs, values, and traditions relating to professionals and organizations, especially health care practitioners and agencies;
- social, class, and geographic boundaries;
- overt and covert mechanisms of oppression and discrimination.

Social and economic history relates, for example, to the availability and quality of employment, schools, and social and health services. A community's beliefs may concern how the community sees its relationship to the external society and/or to other communities. Values and traditions are shaped by the cultural background(s) in the community, which may be homogeneous, but in a rapidly diversifying society may also have differing values and tradition. In the latter instance, efforts to build collaborations or coalitions face possible intracommunity conflicts or tensions. A community is generally understood as having geographic boundaries. However, geographic boundaries may interact with social and economic class boundaries that are less discernable to outsiders, but will have to be considered in community program planning. Last, because ambulatory health care in general, and social work in particular, targets the needs of at-risk populations, consumers with unmet needs—each of which are disproportionately represented in minority populations—oppression and discrimination historically, currently, and potentially in the future are areas of import in understanding communities. Each of these characteristics can ease the process of community-based health care programs, or act as challenges.

Processes for Understanding a Community, Consumer Group, Problem, and Organization

Netting and colleagues (2004) identify a process and specific activities for the practitioner to gain an understanding of populations, problems, and organizations, several of which are pertinent to practice on behalf of health consumer groups (Netting, Kettner, & McMurty, 2004). A practitioner's first step in understanding health care populations, problems, and organizations is an exploration of relevant information. This process involves collection of social and community data and a review of the empirical literature—ideally empirical literature that combines the population and the problem—to gain understanding of the context of the consumer group, problem, community, and the organizations involved. Based on social work's ecological perspective and in pursuit of cultural competence, the following are priorities in this process:

- information and empirical knowledge about the consumer group and the health problem;
- empirical evidence of efforts to resolve the problem, preferably with a similar population;
- the cultural context of the population or group and how that cultural background interfaces with the problem;
- related local history of the problem, efforts to address it, and organizations and/or community constituents involved.

Relevant sources, such as census data and community resource guides, supply demographic characteristics of the population, the problem, and agencies. Several Web sites supply exhaustive amounts of current data on population and community demographics, and health and social indicators. Federal databases are good places to start in general; specifically for community health practice, the U.S. Centers for Disease Control (www.cdc.gov) and the Census Bureau (www. census.gov) are very useful. Federal and state Web sites provide population demographics and health statistics retrievable on state, county, and zip code levels by gender, age, and racial groups (for further sources see Appendix B on Web site summaries). Community resource guides and the worker's own knowledge identify the organizations and community groups related to the population and or problem. Data collection begins to inform the practitioner's ecological perspective of a population and/or health condition or problem and possible associations between consumers, health problems, and socioeconomic conditions.

The literature search expands the census data knowledge and begins the process of furnishing a biopsychosocial context of the consumer group and health condition, and identifying possible effective interventions. These information gathering and literature review processes result in determining

- what is known about the population and the health problem at hand;
- possible relevant evidence-based interventions;
- related cultural background issues;
- local involved organizations, agencies, and community groups.

Interviewing to Expand Understanding of the Context

In addition to having the data to describe a consumer group and problem for planning a program, social workers need knowledge of the context of a project. Knowledge of the context of a community, consumer group(s), and/or problem(s) can be acquired through a particular type of interviewing. Key informant interviews are more akin to ethnographic interviews (i.e., what the situation looks like from this person's perspective) than social work interviews with clients. The purpose of the former is to see the issues from an insider's viewpoints, rather than to assess problems and plan interventions as in the latter. Interviews with key informant organizational and community leaders and members of the consumer population supply the history and the local community context of a consumer group, health issues, and the organizations or agencies involved now and in the past.

Interviewing individuals of the potentially or currently involved organizations and providers can identify organizational decision makers and furnish understanding of the history of current and/or previous interorganizational efforts and funding possibilities concerning the population and health condition of interest. Community resource guides and colleagues can direct the worker to possible organizations of relevance, and identify those recently and currently involved in service delivery to the targeted population and/or health condition. Practitioners are mindful of the characteristics of organizations discussed previously in interviews to assess organizational receptivity to the program and to identify potential issues inhibiting effective interorganizational collaboration. Respect and clear communication about the intent of interviews, with sensitivity for the varying perspectives of key organizational and interdisciplinary professional interviewees, is ethical and eases the way to gaining important information. The pertinent questions directing practitioners in key informant interviews for planning in ambulatory health care practice on behalf of consumer groups are as follows:

- What are the organizations and agencies that provide services to the consumer group and/or health condition?
- What is the structure of the organizations? Who are the key leaders?

- What are the historical relationships among the involved agencies?
- Do the agencies compete for resources or clients of the consumer group?

Put into application the information collection, literature review, and interview process that enlighten planning for an adolescent pregnancy prevention program. In fact, data collection finds that rates of adolescent pregnancy continue to increase throughout the nation and the local community. Higher rates of pregnancy and negative pregnancy and birth outcomes are associated with younger mothers, particularly those aged eighteen and under, and minority group membership (e.g., Mason et al., 2001; Roby & Woodson, 2004). Thus, a pregnancy prevention program for teens in the community might be an area of interest for ambulatory health care social work.

A knowledgeable practitioner engaged in planning the project would then conduct a literature review on teen pregnancy programs and encounter a plethora of studies covering the last few decades— a daunting amount of reading and analysis (e.g., Monahan, 2001). However, further searching would find a recent analysis of outcome studies of teen pregnancy prevention programs implemented in schools and clinics over the last decade across the nation (Franklin and Corcoran, 2000). Counterintuitively, Franklin and Corcoran's conclusions were that clinic-based, rather than school-based, programs were more effective in preventing teen pregnancies. Further, designing educational content by the age and developmental stage of the teen group(s) and basing curricula on social learning theory enhanced effectiveness. The practitioner now would engage in interviews with people from the community, consumer population, and organizations to fill in the local context. Following the leads from empirical findings, the worker would in particular interview clinic providers and personnel.

As a second illustration of the value of a literature review and assessment of cultural context is a study by Hatchett and Duran (2002). As reported in census and Centers of Disease Control and Prevention data, Hatchett and Duran note that Latinas, particularly older adults, are at the greatest risk for HIV infection among all women. Latinas represent one-fifth of all AIDS cases, though they constitute only one-tenth of the overall U.S. population. It is believed that the increased risk may be due to behavioral factors related to culture and religion. In light of these demographic statistics, a community HIV-prevention program for adult, largely Catholic, Latina health care consumers was implemented. Hatchett and Duran note the importance of including the faith community in planning, and giving attention to the Catholic church's HIV prevention approaches, as have others (e.g., Paz, 2000). Further, the Latino culture has specific gender roles and social rules and values concerning sexuality that may influence Latinos' responses to health risks, including HIV infection (Weaver, 2005). Planning ambulatory health care HIV-prevention community-based projects with Latinas would wisely take care of these cultural issues.

In summary, collection of data, review of the empirical literature, and informant interviews inform the social worker of the major issues to be considered and related factors for planning programs on behalf of a consumer group. These processes can also direct attention to the interventions most likely to succeed with the consumer group and/or health condition community-based programs.

CHALLENGES IN INTERAGENCY PRACTICE ON BEHALF OF CONSUMER POPULATIONS

Challenges to community programs for health care consumer populations can arise from characteristics of the organizations, such as those discussed previously, and/or of the consumer group, health condition or risk factor, and/or local history.

Organizational factors that may be challenging can stem, for example, from organizational authority, stakes, and/or interpersonal factors. Agencies may see developing programs to resolve fragmented service systems as potentially resulting in competition over resources, such as revenue from client services, or staff, and lead to turf battles or inertia within the interorganizational group, particularly when bureaucratic organizations are involved (Netting, Kettner, & McMurty, 2004). The challenges arising from the personal and professional factors discussed previously may relate to role status, professional identity, or history. Powell and co-authors note that professional factors that may interfere with effective program planning include perceived "unequal distribution of power" and "professional vulnerability" related to discipline, and/or organizational affiliation

(Powell et al., 1999). Activities that help the organizational participants come to a collective vision of the project and to commit the time
needed for the project are of particular import in overcoming these
challenges (Shortell et al., 2002).

Cultural responsiveness, self-awareness, and "taking the learner's
stance" are just as important in planning for practice on behalf of
populations as in direct practice with individual consumers and their
families. The elements of cultural background discussed in Chapter 3
are applicable to practice on behalf of consumer groups. Knowledge
of culturally related health practices and beliefs of the consumer population is necessary for culturally responsive programs. For example,
how does the consumer group see its role in changing the health condition, and how are allopathic medicine and/or indigenous community healers related? Are there germane relationships with cultural
healers or community centers or faith groups? Are family structures,
roles, and social values of the population interrelated with the health
problem? Is there a need for language interpreters? Are issues of immigration present? Informant interviews guide the practitioner in
planning by answering how the cultural context of this consumer
group relates to the health condition, the group's prior history in programs about this problem, and in identifying representatives of the
cultural communities to be included in planning.

Programs on behalf of culturally diverse or rapidly growing consumer groups, such as immigrant populations, challenge cultural
responsiveness, specifically language compatibility, in engaging consumer participants (Chillag et al., 2002). Social work skills in leadership, group process, and culturally responsive assessment and practice
are crucial in overcoming these challenges. Identifying culturally related values, norms, and health beliefs and practices, and understanding that a cultural group is heterogeneous rather than uniform, as in
direct practice, guides practitioners in the planning and development,
and ultimately implementation, of programs for consumer groups
(Kreuter, Lukwago, Bucholtz, Clark, & Sanders-Thompson, 2002).

As an illustration, evidence suggests that programs in African-
American communities benefit from professionals investing time and
energy to build trust with community groups, and in interagency co-
operation. A history regarding race and socioeconomic class among
organizations can create tensions in conjoint activities (Thompson,

Minkler, Bell, Rose, & Butler, 2003). Social workers know the history of oppression and unethical health interventions in black populations, and they can educate other professionals and agency participants about the impact of this history on constituent participation. A culturally competent lens highlights the history, values, and social structures relevant to African-American communities. As an illustration, inclusion of church leaders in the community is essential in program planning in black as well as other cultural groups. In Latino communities, the value of interpersonal relationships can be reflected by practitioners in supporting mutual processing among professionals, agency representatives, and community members throughout planning and development of community health programs (see also Chapter 3 on cultural background for further discussion).

In brief, knowledge of and the processes for assessing the dynamics and characteristics of organizations, communities, consumer groups and health conditions, and cultural responsiveness in work with diverse groups and communities and the processes for analyzing these provide the basis for practice on behalf of consumer populations.

COLLABORATIONS AND COALITIONS/CONSORTIA

Practice on behalf of consumer groups involves planning, developing, and implementing health care programs in collaborations and coalitions/consortia, or a combination of these strategies. The following discussion explores these approaches, related challenges, empirical findings, and examples of health consumer programs. The discussion incorporates social work skills and concepts as appropriate.

Collaboration

First, a word to clarify two terms: collaboration and coordination. Some confusion exists in the literature on the meaning of the term "collaboration"; it may refer to a method of connecting, or to a type of connection. In this discussion, collaboration is a joint effort of two or more agencies or organizations in planned change to create a new program or service for a population or community. Collaborations in community health care, as in general, share resources communally to create an interorganizational infrastructure(s). In contrast, coordination is defined as working together to assure a continuum of care for consumers, one consumer at a time, through existing services as discussed in Chapter 5 on direct practice. Though the line between these two interpretations is narrow, in the present discussion, collaboration is an approach in ambulatory health programs on behalf of a consumer group, population, or consumers with a health condition or risk factor(s).

What Is Necessary for Successful Interorganizational and Intergroup Collaboration?

What characterizes interorganizational collaboration efforts in community-based health care? In terms of ambulatory health care, interorganizational collaboration most often relates to change(s) needed to resolve fragmentation in care delivery systems, gaps in services, or unmet needs for a population of health care consumers. Collaboration is the strategy of choice in these instances because individual organizations or consumer groups could not resolve the problem on their own.

Certain elements must be present for an interorganizational collaboration to be successful. For example, to resolve a fragmented health care system for adolescent mothers, the organizations or agencies involved in a collaboration should

- share common ground in regard to the consumer population, either by
  1. already serving the population or addressing the health issue;
  2. and/or being committed to serving the consumer group or condition;
- accept that the current service system is fragmented and/or that the consumer population's needs are not met;
- agree that a collaborative interorganizational effort can resolve the problem.

Successful collaborations are not easily or quickly established. Cameron and Mauksch (2002), in a stellar article, report the challenges and methods to overcome the challenges of collaboration. They describe an interorganizational collaboration to integrate community services to meet the mental health needs of the consumers of a single primary care health center that exclusively serves the uninsured population of a county. The challenges encountered reflect the issues noted previously, such as overcoming barriers arising from organizational control, decision making, and authority, and integrating the professional perspectives and cultures of the organizations (i.e., primary care, medical and mental health, community practice). The authors report that these, and other challenges, were overcome ultimately by

- all organizations committing sufficient time for the planning and development;
- studying and assessing the size and needs of the consumer population;
- building on existing professional and organizational relationships;
- ongoing interorganizational and interdisciplinary education and training;
- using empowering tactics, such as having participants do peer training.

A commitment to the time necessary is very important and linked to long-term outcomes of a program, and to getting multiple groups and constituencies to work together (Shortell et al., 2002). In sum, the overall objective of these strategies is the development of partnership relationships among organizations and groups, a requisite in community-based health care collaboration. Social work skills in assessing consumer problems, identifying resources, negotiating among systems, and building on existing strengths are indispensable in cultivating partnerships (Arches, 2001).

Not surprisingly, social work ethical principles and values come into play in health programs for at-risk and disadvantaged consumer populations. For example, involving consumers in planning processes respects diversity, is empowering, and promotes self-determination. As illustrations, two health care programs operationalize social work values and principles in community-based health care collaborative programs for at-risk and disadvantaged health consumer groups.

Bowie and Rocha (2004) describe an organizational-community collaboration to resolve fragmented health care in a community-based program that includes an impressive range of services (e.g., health center, entrepreneurial and business development, training, and child care). The health center has primary care and prevention and wellness components; its 2,000 residents are located in public housing; and it provides comprehensive medical services with a full-time medical and nursing staff. The health and wellness program of the center provide educational, screening, and training programs; prenatal and nutrition classes; and a weight training and sports activity center. Most notably, program planning and development employed empowerment and participatory practice social work strategies. For instance, initial steps in planning included a community needs assessment, and involving community representatives throughout planning and development, as well as building a committed partnership with a local hospital to provide staff.

A second example of successful collaboration is Patch, a typical service delivery model in Britain to address fragmentation and gaps in services, which was transplanted to the Midwest. The Patch approach locates all the services needed by members of a neighborhood within that neighborhood or "patch." Colocation of service providers in one site in the neighborhood of the consumers is the hallmark of the Patch approach. Strategies in development of the family-centered community-based program include creating teams of interagency representatives, residents, professionals, and advocates. Partnerships committed to a project and to changing the status quo of the ways services are traditionally delivered are linked to translating the vision of the program into an evolving reality of the program, attendant policies, and procedures (National Resource Center for Family Centered Practice, 2004).

In aggregate, these two programs represent successful collaborations characterized by the planning and development of an infrastructure to provide care to resolve fragmentation and address the unmet needs of a consumer population. In each program, agencies and organizations contribute resources and staff to a program with their loyalty and commitment moving from the original employer to the project and its consumers. In each program, professionals are colocated in a site within the neighborhood of those it seeks to serve. Last, each program builds upon empowerment and partnership strategies incorporating community representatives, organizational leaders, and consumers in the process. Figure 6.1 depicts a collaborative infrastructure.

Collaborative infrastructures are one approach to resolving fragmentation of health care systems and meeting the needs of at-risk or

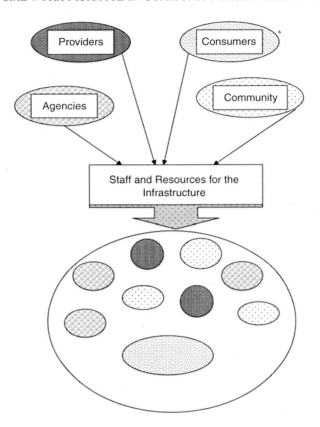

FIGURE 6.1. Collaboration to develop an infrastructure.

vulnerable health care consumers. A second is a network of stakeholders and providers in coalitions/consortia. This approach is the topic of the next section.

Coalitions/Consortia

The second type of interorganizational community-based approach is coalitions or consortia. In this discussion, these two terms are used interchangeably. A coalition is also a collection of organizations and/or consumer groups, but in contrast to collaborations, tends to be more loosely constructed, and to come together for a singular goal, such as an unmet need for service (Dunlop & Angell, 2001). Moreover, the members of a coalition maintain their primary identification outside the coalition, but share commitment to the goal of the group. In traditional form, a coalition ceases upon success in reaching its goal, though it may take on another specific singular goal.

In consortia, agencies or organizations that serve a health consumer population delegate staff members, in common, to the coalition, for instance, to develop a better consumer pathway or to meet a particular consumer need. In this model, sometimes referred to as a network, delegated staff persons remain employees of their respective organizations. Coalitions in community health care characteristically include consumers and agency, organization, and community representatives, each with a variety of interests. Figure 6.2 is a depiction of a coalition or consortia.

While the overt goal of community-based health care coalitions is often to integrate existing service systems, health care consumer participants are empowered in the process (Galambos, 2003; Kreuter, Lezin, & Young, 2000). Empowerment strategies include involving the broadest range of community and consumer stakeholders in the process of planning. Recruiting and successfully involving stake-

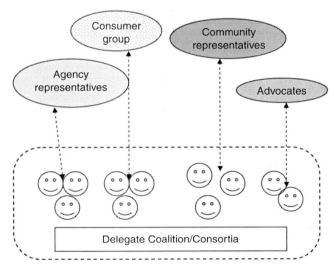

FIGURE 6.2. Coalition/consortia on behalf of health care consumers.

holders and consumers is challenging, and it may raise consideration of concrete needs, such as transportation and child care and leadership training. In addition, depending on the experiences of stakeholders in previous community-based groups, prior history may assist or restrain development of the coalition, as can a history of interpersonal socioeconomic and intercultural tensions. Overall, recommendations for success in involving community leaders and consumers in consortia development in ambulatory health projects are

- having a well-defined, specific issue;
- agreeing upon the mission and goal;
- emphasizing leadership, rather than management.

Empowerment strategies help increase ownership, cultural sensitivity, and feelings of competency, responsibility, and helpfulness among community and consumer participants, and, taken together, these strategies have the benefit of contributing to sustaining and maintaining the coalition (Kreuter, Lezin, & Young, 2000).

Cultural responsiveness is key to effective coalition building in the community. For example, an evaluation of Healthy Start Programs nationally found that cultural responsiveness—seeing the project through the eyes of participants—and the strengths perspective were essential in capacity building in community-based programs (Ramos, & Ferreira-Pinto, 2002; Thompson, Minkler, Bell, Rose, & Butler, 2003). Capacity building refers to activities or methods that increase participation, empower, and develop leadership in communities or community groups. Recommended strategies to achieve these objectives include

- ongoing outreach to consumers and their cultural community;
- offering incentives for participation (e.g., transportation, child care);
- promoting reciprocal interactions among professional, consumer, and community members of the consortia;
- helping consumer groups identify shared concerns and including these in planning;
- training consumers in leadership skills with opportunities to experience leadership roles.

Social work expertise in bringing together culturally diverse groups, and small group processes, though not necessarily known a priori by coalition members, is invaluable in building constituent participation in collaborations and coalitions/consortia; practitioners may often need to intentionally demonstrate these skills (Poole & Van Hook, 1997). Social work skills in spanning the boundaries of organizations, agencies, and stakeholder consumer and community groups are integral in developing and maintaining relationships (Dunlop & Angell, 2001). Boundary spanning skills are the linkage, information processing, and negotiating activities implemented among and between organizations and constituent groups.

In sum, social workers skilled in empowerment, capacity building, and intergroup relationships are influential in resolving the tensions arising among constituent groups and organizations, and the interactions of history, the sociopolitical environment, and the interests of those involved in collaborations, coalitions, and consortia.

HEALTH PROMOTION IN PROGRAMS ON BEHALF OF CONSUMER GROUPS

Collaborative and coalition approaches to resolve fragmentation of health services and to address the unmet needs of consumer groups often employ health promotion and prevention methods.

Health promotion is a holistic approach, traditionally thought of as a public health approach that is linked to quality of life for both individuals and communities; social workers have long been encouraged to utilize health promotion in health practice (Rosenberg & Holden, 1997). With the growing emphasis on wellness and prevention, community-based practice on behalf of health consumer groups increasingly incorporates health promotion. Health promotion is often a primary prevention method—precluding the occurrence of a disease—but may also be used in secondary prevention—deterring the side effects of an existing health condition.

Dziegielewski and Jacinto (2004) describe two overall goals of health promotion with a wellness focus:

- consumers are knowledgeable about risks and benefits of lifestyle changes;
- consumers are motivated to engage in health benefiting behaviors.

Social workers plan and implement primary prevention programs to increase awareness of health risk behaviors in vulnerable consumer populations. Strategies to meet these objectives are educational, incorporating some techniques from the cognitive-behavioral approach. Initial steps in health promotion include education of the risk factors in lifestyle or behaviors that lead to ill health or disease. Cognitive interventions link beliefs concerning lifestyle and behavior changes to health, and continuing risky behaviors to illness, and reinforce the benefits of change. Reinforcement of and repeating information is vital because health behavior change occurs incrementally. Health promotion programs are successful when they are planned well for a specific consumer population; cultural responsiveness is of the essence.

Dziegielewski and Jacinto (2004) offer specific recommendations to build on inclusiveness and empowerment in planning and developing educational materials for health promotion programs. These are

- include consumers in the development of educational materials;
- hand out materials directly to consumers, rather than merely referring to other sources for information;
- ensure that materials
  1. are written appropriately for the population's or group's culture, language, and educational level;
  2. have major points highlighted;
  3. are brief.

Health promotion programs in communities can benefit greatly from marketing strategies. For example, communicating information about health promotion programs to all facets of a consumer population as well as the wider community and the organizations that provide health care to the population is advantageous.

As an illustration, Auslander and coauthors describe developing, implementing, and evaluating a health promotion program for minority consumers at risk for diabetes (Auslander, Haire-Joshu, Houston, Williams, & Krebill, 2000). A discussion of diabetes in Chapter 2 detailed the higher rates of diabetes in African Americans, especially women. A basis for the program was the empirical evidence linking obesity and diabetes, and obesity and lower socioeconomic levels among black women. The elegantly designed program randomly assigned 239 African-American women to intervention and control groups to promote dietary change, health risk awareness, and self-efficacy. Interventions were based on the empirical literature that identifies the relevance of culture-related health and dietary beliefs and obesity in minority populations, and cultural context and inclusiveness in community interventions. Thus, educational groups were peer led; educational materials and cognitive-behavioral interventions were culturally specific and developed with input from focus groups of consumers. Pre/post analyses demonstrated that knowledge of nutrition was significantly increased and dietary fat intake significantly reduced in the intervention group.

In brief, the program and its evaluation discussed by Auslander and colleagues is a demonstration of the content of this chapter on the effective use of the social data, the empirical literature, key informant interviews, and cultural responsiveness in developing and implementing community programs for a consumer group.

LEADERSHIP ON BEHALF OF CONSUMER GROUPS: WHAT MAKES A LEADER EFFECTIVE?

A recurrent theme is evident in this chapter: the necessity that social workers in practice on behalf of health consumer populations are skillful leaders. Practitioners in this area of practice may be formally designated or informally function in the role of leader. In either circumstance and regardless of the type of programmatic approach, effective leaders will effectively cross organizational and community group boundaries and manage relationships with consumer populations, community groups, and organizations.

The literature identifies the ability to envision a future that transcends the status quo and to communicate that vision as characteristics of successful leaders. Effective social work leaders evidence commitment to the *Code of Ethics,* the values of inclusiveness and skills in empowering stakeholders (Rank & Hutchison, 2000). Gellis (2001) identified two types of leadership styles—transactional and transformational. According to Gellis, transformational leaders

- produce change by emphasizing a vision of the future;
- are intellectually stimulating;

- inspire others to set aside their own individual and/or agency interests in deference to the interests of the collective group (e.g., planning group, program, neighborhood, etc.).

Transformational leaders are charismatic and creative; they are actively considerate, respectful of, and skillful in motivating others. Charisma is a complex construct including the ability to arouse passion in others, to articulate a vision with which others identify, to develop goals that reach beyond the everyday tasks of a job or program, and to instill both respect and loyalty. Transformational leaders are creative because they

- are able to understand multiple viewpoints;
- understand and solve problems in unique ways.

In contrast, transactional leadership, sometimes called interactive leadership, is based on a series of exchanges between leaders and followers, using a traditional problem solving and contingent reward approach that tends to focus on mistakes.

In comparing these two types of leaders and leadership styles, leadership in ambulatory health care practice on behalf of consumer populations benefits most from transformational, rather than transactional, leadership. Specifically, initiatives to resolve fragmented health care service systems, to address unmet needs, or to address a health or disease condition by definition involve change in the status quo. Change in the status quo—the normative ways of delivering health care—requires a vision and the ability to inspire others to join in making that vision manifest. Now, admittedly, there are no vitamins to boost up our levels of charisma. On the other hand, inclusiveness is a fundamental social work value, as is respect, because varying viewpoints and diversity are professional ethical obligations. These values reflect the characteristics of transformative leadership. In addition, skills in effective and rapid rapport building and establishing trust, knowledge of communities and organizations, and cultural responsiveness contribute to inspiring others with a vision and instilling commitment. In sum, social workers are uniquely prepared for transformative leadership in health care programs on behalf of consumer groups.

ETHICAL CONSIDERATIONS

First, be assured that practice on behalf of health populations is based on the profession's values and ethical principles just as is direct practice. Ethical dilemmas are not exclusive to direct practice. Rather, social workers in practice on behalf of health consumer groups and populations experience situations with ethical implications or dilemmas, some of which also reflect social work values of equity and social justice (Lowenberg, Dogloff, & Harrington, 2000; Netting, Kettner, & McMurty, 2004).

For example, social work values the autonomy of individuals to shape their own lives; that value is affirmed in the ethical principle of client self-determination. Practice on behalf of consumer groups in community-based health care often incorporates empowerment strategies—strategies based on the value and ethical principle of self-determination—to involve consumers and community members. As noted by Netting and colleagues, practice in the community also extends beyond empowering individuals to attending to the concept of beneficence and social justice for groups and communities. Beneficence in colloquial terms means for the good of all; social justice relates to the equitable (i.e., fair) distribution of goods and services. In addition, therein can reside an ethical conflict in practice with consumer groups or populations.

What if planning and implementing one program for one group of health consumers diminishes access or resources for another group? As an illustration, let us suppose that implementing the program presented in the next section to educate children with asthma and their families in elementary schools necessitated, due to available space, that after-school day care for children with special needs in the schools shorten its hours of operation? That is clearly an ethical conflict about well-being between the two groups and the equitable distribution of limited resources of the two groups.

Health care practice on behalf of consumer populations also can involve *practice* dilemmas. Participation in collaborations, coalitions, and consortia may entail confusion or ambiguity about for whom the practitioner is working. By way of illustration of *practice* dilemmas, activities to recruit and empower consumers may send the message that they are the worker's "captain," while in the process of negotiating and resolving turf conflicts in interorganizational relationships, workers may be perceived as employees of one or another of the agencies.

Practice on behalf of health populations may include ethical conflicts over confidentiality and the ethical obligations to challenge social injustice and to promote the well-being of groups and communities. As an example of confidentiality conflicts, a practitioner learns from one constituent consumer group that some consumers in the program believe they are discriminated against in the planning and development processes. Clearly, disclosing the information to other groups in the project abridges confidentiality and certainly could damage further effective relationships. Commitment to social justice is involved if discrimination is present. How to assure that the project is ethical and socially just while also maintaining confidentiality? One possibility is by supporting the group to take the issue to the wider group.

Practice with multiple organizations and groups can raise an ethical dilemma when, as suggested by Lowenberg and coauthors, a social worker is employed by one of the organizations, but whose role is within the collaboration or coalition. To whom does the worker have primary ethical obligations? Social workers are ethically bound to support the welfare of their employers and clients/client groups. In sum, most authors suggest that the primacy of obligations to consumers supersedes those to employers.

Careful deliberation in these ethical dilemma situations is required. Evaluating the comparative benefits and costs of various resolutions, as in direct practice, is the appropriate strategy, though perfect solutions are rarely possible. Effective implementation of a resolution in collaborations and consortia is likely to depend on the social worker's skills in negotiating conflicts and leadership.

APPLYING THE CONCEPTS FOR LOGIC MODELING OF A COMMUNITY PROGRAM FOR CHILDREN WITH ASTHMA

The purpose of this section of the chapter is to apply logic modeling in planning a hypothetical health promotion program in community health for Latino families with children diagnosed with asthma. By way of background, previous chapters identified

- the increasing prevalence rates of pediatric asthma in general;
- the important role of the family in the child's health and care;
- cultural health beliefs and practices in the care of children with asthma;
- the centrality of religion specifically among Latinos.

Last, a review of the relevant literature indicated the effectiveness of education interventions with parents in controlling asthma attacks, the importance of Spanish in educational materials, and bilingual instructors in community-based programs.

In our hypothetical case, social workers in a family services program in an inner city neighborhood with a high proportion of persons with a Hispanic cultural background noticed the increasing number of Latino children with asthma. The exploration of the literature summarized previously and analysis of social indicator data and community programs corroborated their impressions. Assessment activities indicated that there were ninety-seven Latino families with asthmatic children, nine relevant organizations and community groups, the importance of empowerment and capacity building, and linkages with local Catholic churches in community-based programs for Latinos. Subsequently, key informants were identified and interviewed, supplying information about the agencies and health care providers serving this consumer population, community groups, and organizations. Given the literature, the practitioners included the leaders of the Catholic church located in the neighborhood and cultural health practitioners in interviews. The results are presented in the following simplified logic model problem and goal statements:

> **Problem statement:** The ninety-seven Latino families with children having asthma in this neighborhood have no program providing culturally responsive, up-to-date information and knowledge, or social support in caring for their asthmatic children, resulting in the compromised health status of the children, and daily stress on families.

Goal statement: Latino families with children having asthma in this neighborhood participate in the development and planning of a program that provides culturally responsive, bilingual, up-to-date information and knowledge and peer social support groups, resulting in an improved health status of the children and coping capacities of families.

A breakdown of the problem statement lists the population problems and issues as the need for a community program that incorporates all local constituent groups in culturally responsive (1) planning, (2) development, (3) providing up-to-date information and knowledge, and (4) social support groups. In brief, according to their review of the literature and relevant data, and appropriate Internet sources, the social workers determine that a coalition method is appropriate for this single focus initiative with concerted attention to culturally related health beliefs, family structure, social values, and the role of faith. The section in the logic model for methods and processes to plan and develop this coalition initially lists the following action points/strategies: (1) locate and recruit the relevant agencies and organizations and consumer group members with attention to bilingual fluency and cultural responsiveness; (2) engage and build relationships among all constituents; (3) partner with the neighborhood-located Catholic church leaders and cultural health practitioners; and (4) obtain local funding to cover materials and supplies. The input section lists the following: (1) space for meetings of the coalition; (2) recruiting and educational materials in Spanish; and (3) constituents who are bilingual. The practitioners attend to ethical considerations of self-determination and confidentiality and take note to assess the possible impact on other community programs and consumer groups of this initiative in light of social justice and equity.

The previous summary combines the results of activities to assess communities, health problems and organizations, and local social/health indicator data, and helps determine the appropriate community approach. The resulting, though only initial, logic model indicates the problem and goal statements, and the problem list, methods, and inputs for planning and developing the hypothetical program. Objectives, results, and outcomes are discussed in the evaluation of this program in Chapter 7 on evaluation of practice and programs.

SUMMARY

This chapter examined areas of social work knowledge and skills for creative and effective practice on behalf of consumer groups. Discussions included concepts, such as the ecological and strengths perspectives, organizational and community factors to understand organizations, health consumer populations and problems, and communities. Exploration of the best practices in collaboration and consortia/coalitions included

- relationship building, boundary spanning, empowerment, and capacity building;
- transformative leadership;
- health promotion.

Last, the ethical considerations in practice on behalf of consumer groups were identified, including potential conflicts over consumer confidentiality and well-being versus program and employer well-being, and the values of social justice and beneficence in ambulatory health care practice with consumer groups and populations. In brief, practice on behalf of consumer groups capitalizes on several areas of social work knowledge and skills, and is predicated on social work values of respect for diverse groups, equity, and promoting resolutions to the needs of at-risk and vulnerable populations.

DISCUSSION QUESTIONS AND ACTIVITIES FOR INDIVIDUALS AND SMALL GROUPS

1. Consider a health consumer population that you know is in need of, or access to, a health care program or services due to fragmentation of delivery systems with resultant gaps in services. Links to the problem include changes in the demographics of the population, interagency relationships, restricted coverage for health care, and competition over client-driven revenues. Develop a logic model to plan and implement a program in ambulatory health care to address the need. In the specific, be sure to detail the process activities to contextualize planning, remember to utilize the appropriate Web site summaries in Appendix

B, identify the constituencies to be involved, and detail the related possible ethical considerations.

2. Consider the following scenario: You are an informal, but acknowledged, leader in a collaboration of geriatric agencies, organizations, and consumers providing comprehensive health care and psychosocial services with reduced fees for older adults (aged fifty-four and over) in a senior services center. The consumer population is about two-fifths black, one-third Asian, one-tenth Latino, and one-tenth white. Recently the social workers, who were originally employees of several agencies in the collaboration and now are practitioners in the program, complain that some of their consumers are "revolving door" clients, some of whom may need geriatric psychiatric assessment for possible cognitive impairment, others of whom misuse alcohol with attendant family and health problems. However, these same consumers tend to have limited coverage for these services outside the center and these services would currently have to be provided outside the center. (a) Analyze the pros and cons of the social work leaders' use of transactional and transformative leadership styles in resolving this problem. (b) What are the potential ethical conflicts between self-determination and societal and cultural beliefs about growing older?

GLOSSARY

advocacy: The practice activities targeted at educating, informing, or representing the needs and wishes on behalf of groups or populations of consumers.

capacity building: The activities or methods used to increase participation, empower, and develop leadership in communities or community groups.

coalitions/consortia: Loosely constructed collections of organizations, consumers, and/or stakeholder groups that come together for a singular goal.

collaboration: The activity of organizations, communities, agencies, and constituent community groups working jointly, and sharing resources to achieve a consensually agreed upon goal and tasks.

community: Human system that may be identified by geographic boundaries, or a commonly shared identity, that functions to provide social participation, socializing members, and the production, distribution, and use of services and goods.

health promotion: A holistic approach, traditionally thought of as a public health approach, that seeks to increase knowledge and awareness of health risks to achieve behaviors and attitudes linked to wellness, reduced risk factors, or both.

host settings: Organizations and agencies dominated by professions, authority, decision making, and management other than social work.

interdisciplinary collaboration: Persons of different professions work jointly in an integrated endeavor to develop and implement a plan of care for consumer groups or populations.

primary prevention: The area of prevention activities that seeks to reduce the susceptibility to disease or illness or the social problems of individuals or populations.

public health: The art and science that deals with the protection and improvement of community health by organized community-based efforts.

secondary prevention: Prevention programs that target early detection of diseases or illnesses so that interventions to change behaviors or risk factors before irreversible negative consequences of the disease or illness occur.

stakeholders: Those who are benefited by or "have a stake" in achieving some goal or objective.

wellness: The quality or state of being in good health, especially as an actively sought goal.

Chapter 7

Evaluating Practice and Programs in Ambulatory Health Care

- *Why evaluate practice?*
- *How is direct practice evaluated?*
- *How are programs on behalf of consumers evaluated?*
- *How can a practitioner assure that evaluation is culturally responsive and ethical?*

WHY EVALUATE SOCIAL WORK PRACTICE?

Previous chapters indicated the importance of evaluating health care interventions and programs by managed care systems in disease management protocols and in the social work literature. Zlotnick and Galambos (2004) recently affirmed that the emphasis on evidence-based practice (EBP) is here to stay and is predicated on social work's commitment to consumers' best interests. In a similar vein, Corcoran, Gingerich, and Briggs (2003) indicate that the reasons for evaluation are based first on the profession's commitment to enhance the well-being of consumers and consumer groups, and to make available the best practice possible. As if additional reasons were necessary, both medicine and managed care are adamant—likely for different reasons—on the need to provide evidence-based interventions. In addi-

Social Work Practice in Community-Based Health Care
© 2007 by The Haworth Press, Inc. All rights reserved.
doi:10.1300/5273_07

tion, practice evaluation can substantiate the "value addition" of social work interventions to management and other disciplines in health settings (Auslander, 2000; Rock & Cooper, 2000). Last, though not necessarily obvious, evaluation informs social workers about their own practice, whether directly with or on behalf of consumers, and answers the question, "How might my practice improve?"

The purpose of this chapter is to present an overview of measurements, design, and analysis of evaluation of interventions in direct practice with health care consumers and in community health care programs on behalf of consumer groups or populations and to apply evaluation to an individual health consumer scenario and a program using the logic model technique. The fervent hope is that, in so doing, practitioners in ambulatory health care will find evaluation both feasible and interesting. It is beyond the intent of this chapter to discuss evaluation of practice in depth. Rather, the chapter consolidates relevant concepts and techniques from the current literature on evaluation (e.g., Bloom, Fischer, & Orme, 2003; Netting, Kettner, & McMurty, 2004; Rossi, Freeman, & Lipsey, 1999).

HOW IS DIRECT PRACTICE EVALUATED?

The overall method of evaluating direct practice is the systematic collection of data to establish whether a social worker's intervention worked as planned and to inform the consumer and the social worker about the impact of interventions on the concerns identified in assessment. A single-system design is appropriate for this type of evaluation.

Single-system designs are applicable to individual and family consumers and across interventions, including small group work. Single-system designs have the advantage of being able to be built into practice adaptively to specific consumers in daily practice. Essentially, direct practice evaluation is a way of determining whether meaningful change has occurred because of a plan of intervention.

For example, Rock and Cooper (2000) describe a single-system design in a university–primary care collaboration to demonstrate the value addition of social work in the setting. Single consumers in the setting were screened with rapid assessment instruments (i.e., the Hudson Scales). Nine student practitioners intervened with those consumers identified as having anxiety or depression of levels indicating the need for services over the course of two years. Analysis of single-subject evaluations showed that student practitioners were effective in intervening with the consumers; a 32 percent increase in social work patient contact was found in preproject/postproject analysis.

Most single-system designs in practice are essentially before-and-after designs: an AB design: A (baseline) and B (intervention) phases. The preintervention (i.e., A baseline) phase may at times be difficult to implement since the sooner a health care consumer is seen, the more possible it is to identify the requirements of managed care and to understand the wishes of clients themselves. However, baseline data can be collected retrospectively or reconstructed when meeting to set up an appointment and/or as a part of the initial meeting (Bloom, Fischer, & Orme, 2003). More complex single-system designs include, for example, ABCD designs where the baseline (A) and intervention (B) phases are followed by no intervention (C), and reinstituted intervention (D). In the time-limited settings of ambulatory health care, these may be impractical (Rock & Cooper, 2000). In addition, some interventions, such as information providing/educational interventions, may have immediate effect. In this situation, "pre" session and "post" session measurements for a single-session/meeting intervention can be utilized, thus approximating the AB design.

The first step in designing a single-system evaluation relates to a component of the assessment process as indicated in Figure 5.1 in Chapter 5. That is, identify the condition or issue of concern, which becomes the target of a planned intervention, and how the issue/target is expected to change because of the intervention. Clarity in identifying the objective of interventions and the target is vital; equally vital is critical thought determining that the problem, the intervention(s), the objective(s), and target(s) are logically and conceptually linked. As indicated in this book, habituated practice, lacking those logical linkages, promotes illogical practice evaluation. By way of one truly terrible example, consider the logic of having a consumer— Tequilla—with anxiety about a new diagnosis and having difficulty following a medical regimen using guided imagery and biofeedback as interventions and evaluating the interventions' effectiveness by measuring Tequilla's self-esteem. There is a missing link here.

Both target issues/problems and objectives are described in client terms, and must be observable and measurable in some way. As an illustration, take the same consumer above, Tequilla, who is anxious about a new diagnosis of borderline hypertension and having difficulty implementing the treatment regimen (i.e., increase physical activity and reduce fat intake). The two issues—anxiety and difficulty—are targets. Let us say that the practitioner and the client decide to use a combination of educational and cognitive-behavioral interventions. Objectives should be clearly stated and client centered, and identify who, what, and how the issue is expected to change because of interventions. Therefore, for that consumer, the objectives might be that she (1) feels comfortable about the diagnosis, and (2) is physically active. Next the worker and the consumer agree on how to measure these two issues/targets.

Applying logic modeling, and in reference to Figure 5.2, the box labeled "problem list" would include anxiety about new diagnosis and difficulty in increasing physical activity. Continuing the logic model, the "objective" box would identify, as described earlier, that Tequilla feels comfortable about her diagnosis and is physically active. Now, how would we measure these two targets?

What Data Collection Techniques Are Used in Single-System Designs?

Measurement is a planned process of assigning values, generally numbers, to certain characteristics. Three types of measurement typical of single-system designs are standardized goal attainment, individual rating scales, and client logs. Several criteria should be met by a measurement (Berkman & Maramaldi, 2001; Bloom, Orme, & Fischer, 2003). Collectively these criteria are that the measure

- is conceptually linked to the consumer's problem;
- be supported by empirical evidence that it operates consistently over time and actually measures what it purports to measure;
- is brief, and easily implemented and scored.

Classically standardized measures are used in before-and-after single-system designs, though their more frequent use during the intervention phase is useful when that phase is of sufficient duration.

These scales result in a summative score of the scale's multi-item ratings. The reader is reminded that several standardized measures were discussed in Chapter 5 on direct practice, and the sources for these and other validated measurements are included in Appendix B on Web site summaries (also see Corcoran & Fischer, 2001).

Goal attainment scaling (GAS) is a type of measurement that shows change in relation to intervention objectives, and it is used by consumers between sessions with the practitioner. GAS measurement allows the consumer to self-monitor as well as to provide workers with frequent feedback. A typical goal attainment scale ranges from 1 to 5, with 1 designated as the least favorable and 5 the most favorable outcome. Intermediate numbers represent a less than expected outcome (i.e., 1 and 2), the expected outcome (i.e., 3), and a greater than expected outcome (i.e., 4 and 5). Most important, in GAS the worker and the consumer describe in words the meaning to the client of each number-identified level of the scale. In some discussions, GAS measures are used only for observable behaviors. When there are distinctions between observable and internal measures, the latter is often referred to as a self-anchored rating scale (SARS). In this discussion, a GAS may be for an observable behavior (e.g., weight loss, sleep, physical activity) or an internal state, such as in Tequilla's scenario her worry about a new diagnosis. A separate GAS is developed for each consumer concern/target and objective. In Tequilla's scenario a GAS for comfort with her diagnosis could be as follows:

1 = feels very uncomfortable: "I worry about it all the time."

2 = feels slight uncomfortable: "I worry about it a good deal."

3 = feels fairly comfortable: "I worry about it occasionally."

4 = feels quite comfortable: "I rarely worry about it."

5 = feels exceedingly comfortable: "I never worry about it."

Given that the community health environment is often based on a medical model of service, it is beneficial to include measurements directly related to the medical problems identified. As an illustration, the objective for Tequilla to be physically active relates directly to medical assessment and treatment. A goal attainment scale could be developed for this target, or the client could record the time engaged in physical activity in minutes per day in a log to provide the data.

Last, given the comparative brevity of a patient's episode of care in community health and the number of sessions a social worker may meet with a consumer, follow-up activities via phone are particularly important. Data on postintervention—B phase—can and should be incorporated in follow-up efforts.

Returning to the final component of a logic model, measurement indicates the extent to which an objective is achieved and, thus, the effectiveness of interventions in short-term results (within the near future) and long-term outcomes (in a year or more as appropriate). Continuing with Tequilla's scenario, the GAS measures on comfort, logs of physical activity, and pre- and postintervention scores on the Hudson Clinical Anxiety Scale supply the indicators of results and outcomes of interventions. By way of a reminder, the Hudson Clinical Anxiety Scale has a clinical cut-point of 30; scores above 30 indicate the need for intervention. Complying with the need to identify who, what, how, and when in evaluation leads us to the following, for example, short-term results and long-term outcomes:

> **Short-term results:** Tequilla is comfortable with her diagnosis as indicated by daily GAS scores within ten days and is engaged in physical activity a minimum of fifteen minutes per day within fourteen days. Clinical Anxiety Scale scores at posttest are below clinical cut-point levels.

> **Long-term outcomes:** Tequilla's health status is excellent by physician report and Tequilla completes a marathon run successfully within one year.

How Are Data from Single-System Designs Analyzed?

The data collected through any of the previously described measurement techniques and design methodologies are generally analyzed visually (Bloom, Fisher, Orme, 2003; Nugent, 2000). Visualization by graphing is particularly helpful for the worker, but just as useful for the consumer, in discerning whether the desired change has occurred. Visualization includes bar and line graphing, each of which can easily be accomplished with Excel spreadsheets, and other computer programs; visualizations can, of course, be created by hand.

Though it is outside the scope of this chapter to examine computer technologies for visualization, Figure 7.1 is an example depicting a bar graph of Tequilla's pre/post scores on the Hudson Clinical Anxiety Scale, and a line graph of Tequilla's GAS measures of comfort with diagnosis. Single-system design data can also be analyzed statistically, though that is beyond the intent of this chapter. However, two excellent resources are available for those requiring in-depth details of statistical analysis, as well as techniques for visualizing data in single-system evaluation (Bloom, Fischer, & Orme, 2003; Patterson & Basham, 2005). As shown in Figure 7.1 the interventions were effective in increasing Tequilla's comfort with diagnosis and reducing her Clinical Anxiety score, though her score remained slightly above the clinical cut-point, at posttest.

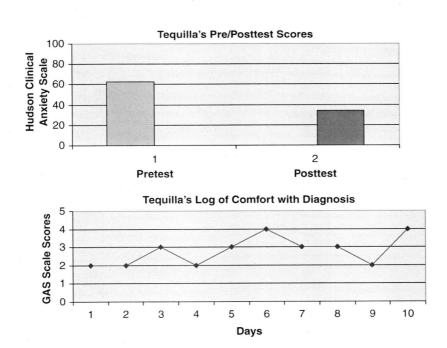

FIGURE 7.1. Bar and line graphs of single-system evaluation.

In summary, the development and implementation of single-system designs makes it comparatively easy to evaluate interventions with individual consumers in ambulatory health care practice. Before-and-after (AB) designs are the most common single-system designs. Appropriate data collected with standardized instruments, goal attainment scales, and consumer logs are analyzed visually; statistical analysis is also possible. The result informs both practitioners and consumers of the efficacy of interventions and may suggest the need for further or different interventions. In brief, single-system evaluation positively contributes to three professional outcomes:

- responding to the mandates of managed care systems for evidence of effectiveness;
- substantiating the value of social work in ambulatory health care practice;
- the ongoing development of individual practitioners.

HOW ARE PROGRAMS IN COMMUNITY-BASED PRACTICE EVALUATED?

Program evaluation includes two types of evaluation in response to two questions. First, process evaluation answers the question, Did the processes to develop the program occur as planned? Second, outcome evaluation answers the question, Did the methods achieve the expected long-term outcomes? That is, in logic model terms, did the methods of planning and development achieve short-term results and long-term outcomes? In program evaluation, short-term results might be seen as the intermediate achievements meeting objectives (mini-goals) and long-term outcomes as attainment of the overall goal. In the context of the discussions in this text on practice on behalf of groups and populations of consumers, this discussion focuses primarily on evaluating planning and development activities, rather than evaluating the effectiveness of a program after it is implemented.

As an example, Chernesky and Grube (2000) describe a process evaluation of case management with HIV/AIDS consumers in three counties in the Northeast. They sought to determine what the influences and elements of case management were across programs to inform determining how to improve programs. Two sources of data were utilized: a purpose sampling of ten charts from each of six agencies that provide case management to HIV/AIDS consumers and focus groups with case managers ($n = 17$).

Results indicated that most clients were contending with multiple psychosocial problems, often regarding concrete issues, (e.g., housing, food), and contacted agencies in times of crisis. Care coordination involved primarily efforts to maintain clients through crises, with inactivity occurring when client crises did not occur. Most important given the multiple needs of this vulnerable population of consumers, interagency boundaries resulted in overlapping use of resources and duplicated efforts for individual consumers. The center of these boundary issues, particularly relevant to the discussions in the previous chapters on fragmented service systems, was found to be that each case manager had his or her own network of resources; resources were not integrated, resulting in redundant client pathways. Barriers to integration included cultural background issues, such as legalities, language, and health beliefs regarding the disease and interacting with physicians, with recently immigrated Latino consumers.

Now let us turn to a hypothesized coalition that was discussed in a previous chapter (Chapter 4) for a community-based program for Latino families with asthmatic children. Taken together, assessment activities found that ninety-seven Latino families in the neighborhood had children with asthma, nine organizations and community groups, one church, and two culturally relevant health practitioners *(curanderos)* were associated with the population. A search of the empirical literature indicated that pediatric asthma prevalence rates are increased in minority groups and associated with negative psychosocial outcomes for the children and family, including increased stress and compromised health status of the affected children. Empirical evidence suggested that effective coalitions are linked to participation that is empowering and capacity building, and culturally responsive. Last, empirical findings suggest that increased knowledge about children's asthma and the availability of peer social support are associated with increased effectiveness in family management of the condition. Consequently, the following problem and goal statements for the coalition were developed:

Problem statement: The ninety-seven Latino families with children having asthma in this neighborhood have no program providing culturally responsive, up-to-date information and knowledge, or social support in caring for their asthmatic children, resulting in compromised health status of the children, and daily stress on families.

Goal statement: Latino families with children having asthma in this neighborhood participate in the development, and planning of a program that provides culturally responsive, bilingual, up-to-date information and knowledge, and peer social support groups, resulting in an improved health status of the children, and the increased coping capacities of families.

Intermediate mini-goals (i.e., objectives) for planning and development would include these, for instance:

- participation of families and community representatives in all planning and development activities;
- inclusion of bilingual participants;
- involvement of representatives from relevant community agencies and organizations;
- mobilization of funds for culturally responsive materials in Spanish;
- development of strategies and activities that are culturally responsive to the consumer population's values, traditions, family structures, roles, and spiritual orientation.

These objectives indicate the short-term expected results of the methods for planning and developing the coalition. Methods include the following:

- recruiting family members, relevant agencies, organizations, consumer groups;
- attending to bilingual fluency of participants and cultural responsiveness in activities;
- engaging in and building relationships among all constituents;
- promoting empowerment and capacity building among family representatives;

- partnering with neighborhood church leaders and cultural health practitioners;
- obtaining local funding to cover materials and supplies.

In aggregate, the evaluation of the processes of planning and developing the program responds to determining how well the methods/interventions led to the achievement of mini-goals. What remains in the process evaluation is to identify what measurements and data collection methods are used.

HOW ARE DATA ANALYZED?

Before exploring data sources and collection, note that this discussion of process evaluation is predicated on the findings of the assessment activities described in a previous chapter substantiating the links between capacity building and empowerment methods, such as recruiting and involving members of the affected families in this program, and achieving effective coalitions. Remember that, as in practice evaluation, measurements must be observable, clearly related to interventions/methods, conceptually linked to the problem, be time-framed, and empirically supported. In addition, the major pothole in determining measurement is that a measurement must address the appropriate unit of analysis. That is, a result relating to utilization of the program that this coalition is developing is not related to the process of development, but is in reference to the program after it exists (i.e., long-term outcome). Data must be collected at the same level at which the intermediate result or the long-term outcome is expected to occur, rather than the reverse.

In process and program evaluation, results and outcomes indicate a time period as well as what the measurements are (Alter & Murty, 1997; Netting, Kettner, & McMurty, 2004). For example, Netting and colleagues (2004) indicate that the initial questions for evaluating process are these: What is the time period for evaluation? What observable measures can be used? Accordingly and in brief, expected results in the evaluation plan for the coalition in this discussion include

- mailings, announcements in organizations, agencies, and the church occur every two weeks within the first two months of planning;
- family participants and organizational and community representatives are recruited within two months;
- representatives from each of the relevant nine community groups, agencies, and organizations and the neighborhood church participate in the coalition within the first three months of planning and development;
- one-third of the coalition members are bilingual;
- the coalition is culturally responsive to the values, social rules, beliefs, and traditions of the Latino cultural background of the consumer group.

Data for these indicators might be collected from attendance notes of coalition meetings, focus groups, interviews, observation of coalition-planning meetings, and/or surveys (Alter & Murty, 1997; Chernesky & Grube, 2000). The cultural salience in deciding what and how data are collected is particularly pertinent to a project such as this coalition. For example, participatory research and qualitative methods are likely to reflect the traditions and values of Latino culture more than quantitative methods (Weaver, 2005). In any case, obviously, linguistic compatibility is essential in those who collect data and the mechanisms (i.e., interviews, focus groups, surveys) of data collection. Of relevance to cultural sensitivity, focus groups are an effective means to get input from those participants most knowledgeable of a particular construct—such as, in this instance, cultural responsiveness (Chernesky & Grube, 2000).

Surveys in the process evaluation could be developed to collect data on the coalition participants' views of the effectiveness of efforts to incorporate bilingual, empowerment, and capacity-building strategies, or cultural responsiveness in planning and development activities. An important point in this activity is to assure that data sources are representative of the full coalition-planning group. In sum, the results indicators answer in numerical terms the following question: To what extent were the methods—recruiting, attending to bilingual fluency and cultural responsiveness, and engaging, building relationships, and partnering—effective in achieving the objectives?

Some also suggest that evaluating resources (i.e., inputs) is a component of process evaluation (Alter & Murty, 1997), while others urge that process evaluation be concerned with experiences of interactions among constituents, not the details of concrete resources (Netting, Kettner, & McMurty, 2004). In compromise of these inconsistencies, consider that the inputs in the logic model for the coalition identify one tangible (i.e., space for coalition meetings) and one intangible (i.e., time commitment) input that, according to the literature, are vital to development.

Evaluating Long-Term Outcomes

Long-term outcomes of the coalition relate to the goal statement. That statement identifies that in addition to the participation of families, a program provides culturally responsive and bilingual up-to-date information and knowledge, makes available peer social support groups, and results in improved health status of the children and coping capacities of families.

Thus, outcome evaluation demonstrates whether the coalition, in addition to being effectively planned and developed as evidenced by process evaluation, achieved instituting the program.

Outcome indicators following the same criteria as detailed previously are expected to occur within a longer time period, usually a year or more. For example, outcome indicators could identify whether

- family participants in the coalition represent a minimum of 20 percent of the ninety-seven Latino families of children with asthma within the first year of the coalition;
- family representatives take on informal and formal leadership roles in the coalition within the first year of the coalition;
- bilingual coalition participants from families and partners from the church and cultural health practitioners engage in developing materials and projects for the program within the first year of the coalition;
- all activities and materials of the program are culturally responsive to the values, social rules, beliefs, and traditions of the Latino cultural background of the consumer group and in Spanish and English.

The measurement of these indicators, and analysis, is similar to the techniques described for collecting process evaluation data.

Evaluation of the program itself, once in place, concerns the effectiveness of the program. Briefly, that evaluation would involve collection of data on the number of program participants, the health status of the children (e.g., attacks, school absences, emergency room visits, and/or hospitalizations) whose families participate, and measures of the stress of families. In addition, interviews and/or surveys of the community on the perception of the cultural responsiveness of the program given the goal would be valuable. Last, in the best of all worlds, evaluation of the effectiveness of the program might involve comparison groups of Latino families that have children with asthma but do not participate in the program.

Analyzing Data in Process and Outcome Evaluations

The techniques for analyzing process evaluation data are largely determined by how data are collected. For instance, quantitative data from meeting notes or surveys are numerically coded and analyzed statistically. In this type of evaluation, analysis is not for the purpose of statistical significance, but to determine if the indicators in the results are achieved. Focus groups and interviews for evaluation purposes are often recorded and transcribed. Analysis of the data from focus groups and interviews requires qualitative analysis to discern patterns and themes reflecting the objectives and the expected results (Patton, 2002). Qualitative analysis is labor intensive. Some computer technologies are available to analyze content more easily (e.g., NUDIST). Outcome measures—the long-term indicators—as is obvious in the previous discussion, are quantitative and quantitatively analyzed.

Ethical Considerations in Evaluation

Though arguments abound as to whether evaluation of practice through any design or methodology is actually research, the profession's ethical code and values are pertinent because evaluation in single-subject designs, process, or outcome evaluations involves consumers and can affect their well-being. Clearly, consideration of self-determination is relevant—Are clients and community members free not to participate in the evaluation? What role may their desire to please evaluators influence their participation and/or data they provide? Is their participation or lack thereof held in confidence?

In coalitions such as the one explored in this chapter, members may be reluctant to fully engage, not from disinterest, but because of prior histories of programs in the community or interpersonal dynamics in the community. As a result, confidentiality and self-determination are crucial values and ethical principles for social work practitioners engaged in evaluation of community-based program development and evaluation on behalf of consumer populations to demonstrate. Social justice and beneficence concerns also arise in evaluation. Does their participation in evaluation influence participants' access to programs or resources? Once again, workers in interorganizational and inter-community group practice are reminded that demonstrating social work ethics and values throughout is recommended to prevent and assist in resolving ethical conflicts should they occur. Leadership skills are beneficial in resolving ethical conflicts among constituent groups and agencies in collaborations and coalitions/consortia.

SUMMARY

To sum up, evaluating the process of planning and development determines whether the methods to achieve short-term objectives were effective and informs how these processes might be improved. Data sources and collection techniques are conceptually linked to the population, the problem, and the objectives in intermediate results. Program evaluation determines whether long-term outcomes are achieved. Cultural sensitivity in the design, measurement, and data collection techniques is pivotal in evaluating social work in community health on behalf of populations and groups of consumers. Last, ethical dilemmas can occur in evaluation and are best prevented and addressed when practitioners are clear about professional ethics and values.

DISCUSSION QUESTIONS
AND ACTIVITIES FOR INDIVIDUALS
AND SMALL GROUPS

1. Develop a process evaluation including short-term results and long-term outcomes for developing a collaborative program to improve the birth outcomes of teen pregnancy in a community with high rates of complicated teen pregnancies and poor health outcomes for both mothers and infants in that population. There are seven programs existing in the community that provide either medical care or home-based postbirth education programs. Several churches of varying faiths, and a mosque, exist in the neighborhood. Consider that the population of teens is largely African American, and most teens are in single-parent homes.
   a. How would your process evaluation attend to cultural sensitivity? What specific elements of cultural background would you consider most important in the evaluation?
   b. How would your process evaluation differ were the target population adults who recently emigrated from Southeast Asia?

GLOSSARY

consumer log: An organized record with which consumers self-monitor behaviors, feelings, or events of relevance to identified problems and issues.

goal attainment scales (GAS): Scales developed collaboratively by consumers and practitioners that are client-centered and that incorporate the goal of interventions with less than expected and greater than expected outcomes in client terms, generally with numbers attached to these levels.

individualized rating scales: Very similar to goal attainment scales, with the main difference being that no requirement that the expected outcome of intervention be the middlemost level.

measurement: The process of assigning values to characteristics; characteristics include, for instance, experiences, feelings, perceptions, or events.

outcome: The expected result of one or more interventions; in this chapter outcomes are long-term indicators of interventions, activities, or methods.

posttest: A measurement that occurs after intervention(s).

pretest: A measurement that occurs before intervention(s).

single-system design: A method for observing change in a single system (e.g., person, couple, family, or small group) over time with systematic, repeated measurement.

standardized scales: Multiple items that have a consistent structure across items, collectively tap a construct or constructs (e.g., feelings, attitudes, behaviors, cognitions), are validated empirically to operate the same across multiple administrations with various groups (i.e., reliability), and actually measure what they are purported to measure (i.e., validity).

APPENDIXES

Appendix A

Exemplars of Innovative Programs in Ambulatory Health Care

BACKGROUND

The following discussion presents four programs that apply the practice approaches presented in this text, respond innovatively to the unmet needs of specific at-risk consumer populations, and include social work services and practitioners. Each exemplar begins with a brief summary of relevant literature.

REACHING OUT TO LATINAS: CULTURAL COMPETENCE IN AN AMBULATORY HEALTH CARE PROGRAM

The Latino population is the fastest growing cultural group in the country (U.S. Census Bureau, 2001). For Latino health consumers, barriers to health care access are multiple, including an increased likelihood of living in poverty, language, and an absence of culturally responsive programs. The following small group intervention in a community health clinic is exemplary for the planning and structuring of the intervention, and in particular for the thoroughness of its cultural responsiveness in the development, implementation, and, particularly, evaluation of the intervention.

These factors are of particular note for Latinas who have the highest rates of fertility of any population group (Roby & Woodson, 2004). As noted by Roby and Woodson (2004), demographic and cultural factors, separation from extended families, and a lack of health care coverage for recent émigrés may explain the low rate of breast-feeding among Latinas, in spite of its well-documented benefits, and increased use by low-income

Social Work Practice in Community-Based Health Care
© 2007 by The Haworth Press, Inc. All rights reserved.
doi:10.1300/5273_08

women of other population groups. The authors note that empirical findings indicate that the single most important factor in the intention to breast-feed among Latinas is prenatal encouragement.

In light of the literature, and a sizable Latino community population, a multidisciplinary group, including social workers and community health workers, developed and implemented a three-session educational intervention program on breast-feeding with a bilingual instructor for Latinas in a western state. Roby and Woodson (2004) describe outreach efforts; strategies included announcement materials at the social services offices, public health clinics, mailings, and personal contacts. In addition, the program provided incentives to participate in all three sessions, and to cover transportation costs to the sessions. The reader is referred to Roby and Woodson (2004) for detailed descriptions of the educational curriculum. The evaluation of the program intervention was well-planned with pre/post measures of participants' knowledge, attitudes, and willingness to breast-feed; measurement tools were in Spanish, validated through pilot testing and reverse translation methods, and implemented by bilingual trained volunteers. Findings suggest that the intervention increased knowledge and the intention to breast-feed, and decreased cultural and myth-based attitudes about lactation.

CREATIVELY RESPONDING TO THE NEEDS OF HIV/AIDS-AFFECTED CHILDREN

The AIDS epidemic has a disproportionate impact on minority cultural groups; nearly two-thirds of those with AIDS are black, Latino, or Asian (Centers for Disease Control, 2001). AIDS is the third leading cause of death among minority women aged twenty-five to forty-four (Winston, 2003). HIV infection and AIDS for minority women is a triply stigmatizing combination of race, gender, and a socially stigmatizing disease and, thus, is associated with social isolation, barriers to services, fear of disclosure, and concerns about child care (Letteney & LaPorte, 2005; Owens, 2003). The following response to the unmet needs of minority women with HIV or AIDS exemplifies creativity and community-based practice in ambulatory health care.

In one county in a southern state, adult women are the fastest growing group of AIDS patients in the state. Given the startling local statistics, the literature, and a two-year community-based research study, the community's Junior League responded in 1994 with a very creative family-centered program. The program, "because no child should be without hope," is called Hope House, a day care center for HIV/AIDS-infected or -affected children, one of only a handful of such programs in the nation (Hope House, 2005, p. 1).

All children at Hope House have a parent with, or who has died from, the disease; of the parents, the majority of whom are African Americans, one-half are mothers, with the remainder largely grandmothers. Hope House provides full-time child care, programs to address children's psychoemotional and physical needs, daily medications, developmental screening, short-term respite care so that parents can attend to their own medical needs, assessment, referral, and follow-up to outside community agencies and resources. Children engage in play therapy while in day care through a partnership with a family service agency. Activities to reduce social isolation and to empower parents include engaging parents in social worker–nurse led social support and educational groups, and in children's educational planning.

Staff includes social workers, nurses, and volunteers who are collaboratively involved with consumer participants in program development and planning. In addition, staff trains public school personnel, health providers, and staff of other day care centers across the community on HIV/AIDS, affected children's needs, and universal precautions.

PARTICIPATORY PROGRAM DEVELOPMENT IN PERINATAL COMMUNITY CARE

Rural health consumers, though representing a small proportion nationally, face a combination of barriers to health care due to combined economic and ecological system factors. Proportionately more rural consumers are uninsured or have only limited coverage compared with urban areas (Centers for Disease Control, 2002). Rural areas have fewer health care providers overall, prenatal care providers in particular, inadequate transportation, and fragmented care systems, characteristics that are risk factors for low birth weight and complicated deliveries (Ginsburg, 2005; Centers for Disease Control, 2002). Recommendations for resolving fragmentation and barriers to maternal health care include colocating psychosocial and health care and involving community providers (e.g., Cunningham & Zayas, 2002).

According to Pistella, Bonati, and Mihalic (2000) and reflecting the literature, over one-quarter of pregnant women in one rural county in a northeastern state with significantly low numbers of primary care and obstetric physicians, and no community health clinics or centers, or transportation resources, delayed prenatal care. Delightfully, however, health, government, human service leaders, community groups, and social workers developed a task force to involve pregnant women and their families in a community-based coalition to gather data and make recommendations to resolve inadequate and fragmented prenatal care. Strategies included involving maternal health consumers in focus groups, needs assessment of perceived barriers to maternal health care to guide planning, and advisory groups with social work leadership facilitating empowerment and capacity building. The consumer needs assessment substantiated that pregnant women who perceived greater barriers significantly delayed prenatal care, and indicated that access to pediatric care, prenatal costs, and social support services for teen mothers were the most serious inadequacies in care.

The program evidences the role of ambulatory health care social workers as leaders on behalf of consumer populations, with expert skills that cross organizational and constituent group boundaries, and empower and build capacities of at-risk health care consumers.

A VISION OF HEALTH CARE FOR THE UNINSURED, WORKING POOR MADE MANIFEST

The number of the uninsured in the United States steadily increases; over 45 million are now without health insurance, disproportionately comprised of minority groups, and with the South having the greatest proportion (20.2 percent) among all regions of the country (Centers for Disease Control and Prevention, 2002). The uninsured are in significantly poorer health and less likely to get health care when needed than those with health care coverage (Van Loon, Borkin, & Steffen, 2002).

The early history of health care management and delivery in the United States targeted the poor and low-paid employees, often spearheaded by single individuals. The Church Health Center reflects this heritage in a faith-based community program to provide comprehensive health care to the working poor and the homeless in the southern United States. The center is the vision of its founder, a physician and ordained Methodist minister, Dr. Scott Morris. Economic and social data indicated that the metropolitan area had a substantial and persistent economically poor and uninsured population, estimated at 150,000 persons.

Community involvement in the development of the center included churches, temples, and mosques; health care providers and hospitals; community groups; and local foundations. The center became operational in 1987 by volunteer physicians and nurses. Church Health now has over 40,000 patients of record, routinely receiving comprehensive care from on-site staff and volunteer physicians, dentists, optometrists, nurses, and social workers and part-time psychiatrists, addiction specialists, and pastoral counselors; on-site radiology and laboratory services are included. In addition, specialist physicians volunteer to offer care when needed in their own offices off-site. Patients can receive medications at the center because local physicians and hospitals donate pharmaceuticals and medical supplies weekly. The center does not utilize any faith-based federal funding sources. A consumer must be either homeless or employed at least part-time and be without a health coverage benefit.

Graduate level, licensed social workers offer comprehensive psychosocial assessments, short-term counseling, care coordination, and staff training, and they collaborate with a community volunteer network for senior companion services, and with a community college in a career development program for clients.

The vision of the center extends beyond comprehensive health care into disease prevention and wellness in its Hope and Healing Center, partially funded by a Robert Woods Johnson grant. Hope and Healing Center facilities consist of a wellness program for weight loss/control, wellness and nutrition education classes, exercise activities and yoga for consumers across the lifespan, physical therapy and a meditation center; membership cost ranges from $15 to $45 for individuals and from $21 to $60 for families, each based on a sliding scale.

Last, the quandary of employees, who make too much to qualify for public coverage, and whose employers cannot afford to provide traditional health care coverage, became clear to the center. In response, Church Health operations include a cooperative plan for the self-employed and employers with fewer than 200 employees to sponsor employees ($10 per employee per month) with an employee share ($45 per month); employee eligibility requirements are minimal, such as having no public health insurance. The plan provides for traditional primary care with an assigned physician and hospital, and includes laboratory testing and dental care; community professionals donate services in their own offices.

In sum, the day-to-day services of the Church Health programs address the unmet health and psychosocial needs of a large, and growing, health care consumer population in ongoing innovations in community partnerships that capitalize on volunteering, whether that be in the time of community persons, supplies, or services.

Appendix B

Web Sites for Social Work in Community-Based Health Care

While there are virtually endless numbers of Web sites on the Internet related in some way to community-based health care practice and consumers, there is also wide variability in their quality, scientific basis, and utility for ambulatory health care. The following summaries of Web sites are the result of a critical analysis of many ostensibly worthy sites for health care, health conditions, and/or social workers in community-based health care practice. The criteria for inclusion were an established organization as sponsor; evidenced-based information; ease of use; content in multiple languages; easily understood glossaries; interactive components for consumers; content for culturally diverse practice and consumers; online support groups; and provider-finding capability. The Web sites included in this appendix met most, if not all, of these criteria. When a Web site met the criteria, but included a particular singular weakness, a *caveat* of that weakness is included in the Web site summary in *italics*.

The Web sites are grouped under the following headings: general health/health condition information; specific disease conditions; major health care organizations; health and minority populations; maternal-child health; the human genome project; and Web sites specifically for social workers.

GENERAL HEALTH TOPICS AND INFORMATION

www.healthfinder.gov

The U.S. Department of Health and Human Services sponsors this Web site that offers information on a variety of health issues; the site is reputed to be the major Web site utilized by the public for health information. The home page offers links for a health library, a "just for you" section, a health

Social Work Practice in Community-Based Health Care
© 2007 by The Haworth Press, Inc. All rights reserved.
doi:10.1300/5273_09

care section, and a directory of health care finder organizations. The Web site speaks directly to consumers in an easy-to-read format. The Web site does not offer a chat room; however, it does have support group listings for various health diagnoses, such as Alzheimer's, lung cancer, or eating disorders, and sections for subpopulations, including individuals at all stages of life, specific racial and ethnic groups, parents, and caregivers. The site is offered in Spanish as well as English, and although it does not include a glossary, it does include a health library with direct links for terms related to prevention and wellness, diseases and conditions, and alternative medicine. The Web site can link users to resources for specific providers in the user's geographical area. There is a subsection specifically for health care professionals that provides information on medical schools, medical errors, funding sources, continuing education, and so on.

www.webmd.com

WebMD offers an exhaustive amount of information on health issues. The home page of WebMD directs individuals to one of four different areas: for consumers—WebMD; for professionals—Health, Medscape, WebMD business services, and WebMD practice services; offered *only in English*. The information provided for consumers is through WebMD health. *Though the Web site may be widely used by consumers, certain subsections warrant professional guidance: a symptom checker; quizzes to assess the likelihood of a particular illness; a drug and herb glossary.* The site has chat rooms focused on numerous health care topics, online message boards, and support groups for over fifty health issues, and subgroups such as the elderly, children, men's health, women's health, and the like. There is a glossary of drugs, health conditions, and a link to locate practitioners.

www.nccam.nih.gov

The Web site of the National Center for Complementary and Alternative Medicine, sponsored by the National Institutes of Health, provides definitions and discussions of alternative and complementary medical (CAM) approaches that are "not presently considered part of conventional medicine." The site includes subsections with information on clinical trials, news releases, a medical dictionary, major categories of alternative treatments and by treatment and disease type, the organization's role and focus, statistical reports of the prevalence of CAM use by treatment category and population groups. The site includes links to find a CAM practitioner, and is available in Spanish. The site provides updated information with documentation references and the basics of alternative medical approaches. *Effective use of some areas would require either knowledge of medical language or use of a medical dictionary.*

www.hhs.gov/ocr/hippa

The U.S. Department of Health and Human Services sponsors this Web site detailing all components of HIPAA of 1996; the site is updated routinely as components of HIPAA are developed and instituted. Links are included on regulations concerning practice guidelines for individual health data acquisition and use; public health data acquisition and use; confidentiality; and transmission of medical records. The site is intended for professional use; the site overall and the glossary are written in professional language only.

SPECIFIC DISEASES OR HEALTH CONDITIONS

Alzheimer's Disease

www.alz.org

This Web site is sponsored by the Alzheimer's Association. The home page offers information on Alzheimer's disease, resources, services, current research, and advocacy and links to the Alzheimer Association's Public Policy Forum, how to make a donation, how to talk to your legislators, and volunteer and career opportunities. The site has subsections for persons affected with Alzheimer's disease, caregivers, and health care professionals, including a chat group and a message board and a comprehensive glossary of relevant terms. The Web site is offered in Spanish as well as English. Many of the links have the option to increase the size of the text for the vision impaired. There is no listing of local providers, but the Web site does offer a 24/7 contact hotline that can provide information on local services.

Amyotrophic Lateral Sclerosis (ALS)

www.alsa.org/resources

This Web site is sponsored by the ALS Association (ALSA) and is included in this appendix because it exemplifies very high quality in health-related Web site geared to consumers and consumer families. Sublinks provide information on caregiving, a travel resource guide, palliative care and grieving, and resources for consumers, such as assistive augmentative communication devices, ramps, personal care aids and wheelchairs, and lift systems to aid in daily living. The Web site includes fact sheets, a patient services resource directory, informative Web links, and a glossary. The site is written with consumers in mind and also includes a sublink for health professionals. The site is only in English and does not include an online chat room or support group. However, the site does include a sublink for locating ALSA affiliates within specific, user-keyed-in locations by state and zip code.

Asthma

www.aaaai.org

The American Academy of Allergy, Asthma & Immunology sponsors this Web site. The home page links include both professional and patient and consumer information, as well as media and subsections. Up-to-date information on asthma, asthma clinical trials, and asthma medications are for professionals; of particular note, is a subsection specifically for patients and consumers that includes online tools, a comprehensive Allergy and Asthma Medication Guide (with downloadable/printable information pages), a link to find medical providers, an extensive glossary of allergic conditions, a subsection to search by condition, and a just for kids section. The latter includes interactive educational games arranged by age, a parent guide, and online ordering of materials. All of the site and subsections are available in Spanish. A best practices section is available for professionals for purchase and includes chapters such as, "Epidemiology," "Barriers to Care," and "Interventions." A separate section, managing the child with asthma, includes assessment, monitoring, and patient education handouts that can be purchased ($10) and copied for educating an asthma patient's caregiver, adolescent patients, and for day care and school staff. Of particular relevance for practitioners are sections concerning establishing school-based programs, including an Asthma Assessment Questionnaire, and suggestions for program development and management.

Cancer

www.cancer.gov

This Web site of the National Cancer Institute (NCI) is sponsored by the U.S. National Institutes of Health. The home page offers links to cancer topics, clinical trials, cancer statistics, research and funding, and news. The Web site has a professional level of information offering current information and the results of clinical/empirical studies that have been done in the area of cancer. There are sections for subpopulations including childhood cancers and women's cancers. The Web site is offered both in Spanish and

English. It also offers a comprehensive glossary that has thousands of cancer terms and provides easy-to-understand definitions. The Web site does not offer chat rooms nor information on support groups and does not link consumers to providers. However there is a section to help consumers learn how to locate providers as well as a phone number for the NCI.

www.cancer.org

This is the American Cancer Society (ACS) Web site. The home page has links for patients, families and friends, survivors, health information seekers, ACS supporters, and professionals. The patients, families and friends, survivors, and health information sections all contain information written on a consumer level and a section for children about coping with cancer. The site is available in Spanish and English; the large glossary of cancer-related terms is in a format that can be easily read. The Web site has an interactive link that helps consumers locate resources in their area; supporter and professional sections are written on a professional level. There are on-site support groups for individuals diagnosed with cancer and an on-line chat support group for cancer survivors.

Cardiac Diseases

www.americanheart.org

The American Heart Association (AHA) Web site provides information on heart disease and strokes. The home page has links for heart disease and stroke warning signs, the American Stroke Association, diseases and conditions, children's health, cardiopulmonary resuscitation (CPR), healthy lifestyle, advocacy, fund raising, publications and resources, news, science and professional information, a heart and stroke encyclopedia with information on hundreds of health issues, local information, and a subsection for children's health. The Web site also provides specific information for health care professionals and provides access to several medical libraries. Information is presented in a format that is easy for consumers to navigate and utilize; however, no chat rooms, support groups, or listings of providers are offered. The AHA Web site is provided in English and Spanish.

www.strokeassociation.com

The American Stroke Association Web site is sponsored by the AHA (see previous entry). The purpose of this site is to provide information on cerebral-vascular accidents, more commonly known as "strokes." The home page has links on warning signs and education on strokes, life after a stroke, a link for health care professionals, a comprehensive encyclopedia of relevant terms, links to online support groups as well as how to start a support group in a user's geographic area, and a media link, but does not include provider lists. The Web site is geared toward both consumers and professionals. The majority of the site is in English only; however, there is a Spanish link offering some information.

Diabetes

www.diabetes.org

The American Diabetes Association (ADA) sponsors this Web site. The home page has links on diabetes prevention and research, nutrition and exercise, and advocacy and community programs. The majority of the information on the site is directed toward consumers, with a vast amount of printable/downloadable information, such as how to choose a blood glucose meter, and the "ups and downs" of using an insulin pump (i.e., the sublink   www.diabetes.org/for-parents-and-kids/diabetes-care/BGMeter.jsp). The Web site includes information on diets and cooking for types of cuisine; ethnic foods and eating at restaurants; and an online store for purchasing resources and books. Within the community programs link there is information specifically for racial and ethnic groups (e.g., diet, lifestyle). The site offers a large portion of its information in Spanish. The Web site does not offer a chat room or a glossary of terms or listings of providers, but it does have a message board allowing consumers to share information. The site includes a link for health professionals that offers information on clinical practice recommendations, professional meetings, current journal articles, and research.

HIV/AIDS

www.aidsinfo.nih.gov

This Web site is sponsored by the U.S. Department of Health and Human Services and provides information about AIDS. The home page of the Web site offers information on AIDS education, resources, news, guidelines, drugs, vaccines, and clinical trials. The information for consumers and providers is written in an appropriate format for each respective group. The information for patients includes information on HIV complications, HIV treatment, caregiving, and insurance/drug assistance. A chat room is offered with live help to answer AIDS-related questions. The Web site is offered in Spanish as well as English and includes a user-friendly glossary explaining many AIDS-related terms. There is no link to help consumers locate providers. Information provided for professionals includes cultural and gender resources, management of HIV complications, maternal-child transmission, and treatment consultation.

Multiple Sclerosis

www.msfacts.org

The Multiple Sclerosis Foundation (MSF) sponsors this Web site offering links for multiple sclerosis information, programs and events, online services, publications, donations, and health care professionals. The information is directed toward consumers and written on a consumer level, but also has information for providers. The Web site has online support groups at specific times; the times are posted and MSF will e-mail a reminder for the chat if given some minimal information. In addition, a support group directory can link consumers with live support groups in their area. The MSF Web site is offered in both English and Spanish; no glossary is available. There is a link to aid consumers in locating an appropriate provider to match their needs.

www.nmss.org

The National Multiple Sclerosis Society (NMSS) sponsors this Web page. The home page offers information on multiple sclerosis, treatments, research, headlines, and special events. The Web page offers information that is easily accessible to clients, but also has a section specifically laid out for professionals. The site offers a chat room link for individuals affected by MS to link to for support. There are sections with information for subpopulations, such as caregivers, teens, and children, and an activity book for children and parents that can be used interactively online or printed and completed offline. The Web site is only offered in English. There is a glossary of terms in lay language in the treatments link; and a listing of treatment locations by state with recommendations on choosing a provider.

Organ Donation and Procurement

www.organdonor.gov

This Web site is sponsored by the U.S. Department of Health and Human Services to provide information on human transplantation, organ donation and organ procurement, policy updates, pending legislation, and statistical data. The obvious purpose of the site is to encourage organ donation and educate concerning the myths and facts about transplantation. The site includes national and state-by-state listings of organizations for organ procurement, organ donation by organ (i.e., kidney, liver, tissue, etc.) categories. There are no chat rooms, and the site is in English only.

Women's and Maternal-Child Health

www.4women.gov/owhpub/minority/index.htm

This Web site is sponsored by the Office on Women's Health of the U.S. Department of Health and Human Services. The Web site includes overall health statistics of women; racial and ethnic groups of women; extensive and well-documented downloadable reports on women's health; health risks and health status. A user-friendly glossary is included, but it is written in a formal style using sophisticated, professional language. The major usefulness of the site is its reports that analyze and compile multiple statistical databases in concise and understandable terms. The site is for informational and professional use, has no links for provider locating, nor for chat rooms/support groups, and is available in English and Spanish.

www.cmchswe.umaryland.edu/health_course_modules

This Web site is sponsored by the University of Maryland School of Social Work offering modules on maternal/child health for social workers developed through multiyear Maternal Child Health, DHHS grant funding. The central theme of the modules is social work with a public health perspective to increase social work students' familiarity with basic concepts of public health. The home page describes the health modules, their purpose, and is for professional use in the classroom. Two categories of modules are offered: Ethnicity and Maternal and Child Health Care; Public Health Perspectives in Maternal and Child Health. Within each module group are several sections, or submodules (e.g., ethics, cultural diversity). The submodules offer a comprehensive explanation of their topics as well as lecture, reading, and discussion question materials for the classroom. As an illustration, within the Public Health Perspectives in Maternal and Child Health is a module on Childhood Asthma that includes annotated bibliographies on the background, epidemiology and risk factors, secondary prevention interventions, and interactive activities to help social workers/students understand the disease and school- and home-based control programs. Many of the modules offer glossaries in an easy-to-understand language. The information is only provided in English; there are no chat rooms, support groups, or links for locating providers.

www.mchb.hrsa.gov

This site is sponsored by the U.S. Department of Health and Human Services for the Maternal and Child Health Bureau (MCHB). The home page has links to information about the bureau, programs, funding opportunities, data, resources, and publications. The information provided is extensive and on a practitioner level, though it pertains to issues of consumers. The site is in English only. The MCHB Web site does not offer a glossary of relevant terms, chat rooms, support groups, or a listing of providers.

MAJOR HEALTH CARE ORGANIZATIONS

www.ama-assn.org

The American Medical Association (AMA) sponsors this Web site offering information for physicians. The home page offers information for becoming a member, AMA agenda, current news, professional resources, and medical schools and residency programs. The information provided is most useful to professionals. The Web site is specifically directed to meet the needs of doctors. The site does not offer a chat room or support groups. It does offer information for doctors in various stages of their career in the member center including medical student section, resident and fellow section, young physicians section, Women physicians, and Congress. The Web site is only in English; no glossary is provided. The site does offer a searchable database for locating physicians by name, location, and specialty. The information that is provided for each doctor is extensive, including office location, office phone and fax numbers, gender, medical school, residency training, hospital admitting privileges, primary specialty, secondary specialty, major professional activity, and other pertinent information. Some doctor information even includes office hours, whether or not the physician is accepting new patients, and what health care plans the physician will accept.

www.amfar.org

The American Foundation for AIDS Research (AMFAR), a major AIDS research funding organization, sponsors this Web site. The home page includes links for information about AIDS research, prevention, education, and advocacy, and is for professionals. The Web site does not offer chat rooms or links to support groups, does not include a glossary or directory of providers, and is only offered in English.

www.apha.org

This Web site is sponsored by the American Public Health Association (APHA). The home page provides various links that are helpful in navigating the site and provide extensive information on, for example, APHA, legislation, advocacy and policy, and public health. The information is intended for health care professionals. The Web site offers an online discussion group for professionals; however, you must be a member of APHA to access this feature. Under the public health links section are subsections for the aging, children's health, gay and lesbian health, men's health, minority health, and women's health. The site is offered only in English and does not include a glossary of terms or sections to search for providers.

www.cdc.gov

The Centers for Disease Control and Prevention, the sponsor for this Web site, is a federally funded organization through the Department of Health and Human Services. The home page has links for health and safety topics, publications and products, and data and statistics. All of the information provided is useful for consumers; however, the detail of the some of the information would be more suitable for professionals. Each link on the home page brings the user to a page where you can search by topic. The information offered on each topic is comprehensive; most of the information includes the most recent results from research performed by the CDC. There are indirect links to subpopulations. The Web site is offered in multiple languages, such as English, Spanish, Chinese, Korean, French, Dutch, Tagalog, Vietnamese, Italian, and Russian. The site also offers an A-Z index with direct links for hundreds of topics. The Web site does not offer a link for consumers to locate providers, chat rooms, or support groups.

HEALTH AND MINORITY POPULATIONS

www.apiahf.org

The Asian and Pacific Islander American Health Forum offers this site sponsored by the U.S. Department of Health and Human Services Office of Minority Health. The home page has links for information on policy advocacy, programs, resources, the organization, ways to support the organization, special events, discussions, a message from the president, and a site map. This site would be useful for any individual interested in learning about advocating for the Asian and Pacific Islander populations. The Web site offers several free-of-charge subscriptions for online groups that exchange information and ideas on various issues facing the Asian and Pacific Islander populations in America. Some portions of the Web site are offered in other languages; however, an individual would need a good command of the English language to find these sections. The site offers information for various groups including Cambodians, Chamorro, Chinese, Filipino, Hmong, Japanese, Koreans, native Hawaiians, Samoans, South Asians, and Vietnamese. The site does not have a glossary of terms or listings of providers.

www.cossmho.org

The National Alliance for Hispanic Health provides this Web site specifically designed to promote the "health and well-being of Hispanics." The home page offers current legislation, resources, and community news that is relevant to the Hispanic population. The information could be useful to consumers or professionals, though most of it is on a professional level. There are no chat rooms or support groups offered for consumers; however, the Web site does offer phone numbers for two bilingual help lines. The site has a large portion of its information in Spanish, although the home page has very few links written in Spanish. The Web site does not offer a glossary of terms, but does have a link connecting consumers with other relevant agencies.

www.ihs.gov

This U.S. Department of Health and Human Services Web site for Indian Health Services (IHS) encompasses the federal health programs for American Indians and Alaskan natives. The home page has a variety of links including jobs and scholarships, medical and professional programs, and nationwide programs and initiatives. Most of the information provided is intended for consumers, though it is also useful for practitioners. The majority of the information is written on a professional level; there are no chat rooms or support groups offered, but the site does offer a section on women's health issues. The Web site has some links in Spanish and others for specific First Nation tribes; the site includes an easily understood glossary of terms and phrases, including indigenous health care terms. The site provides a link for individuals to find resources/providers offered in their geographic area through the IHS.

www.omhrc.gov

This is the Web site of the U.S. Department of Health and Human Services, Office of Minority Health. The home page offers links for new information, initiatives, programs, health disparities, and a resource center. Most of the information is on a professional level, though the information itself may be more relevant for consumers. No chat rooms, links to support groups, or glossary of pertinent terms are provided on the Web site. There is a subsection of information for consumers with HIV or AIDS in Spanish and English and a Resource Persons Network for providers to ask questions to better serve the minority populations.

GENETICS

www.cancer.gov/cancertopics/pdq/genetics/risk-assessment

This Web site is offered by the National Cancer Institute (NCI). The site contains the most up-to-date information on genetic predispositions/factors for cancers and is available in extensive overview sections, and for specific cancers. The site includes links on decision making for genetic testing, and related factors for consideration that are helpful for consumers and practitioners. Links specifically for practitioners discuss basic information on genetics and genetic testing, elements of cancer genetic risk assessment and counseling, counseling about risk factors and risk management, the psychological impact of genetic information and testing for the individual and the family, posttest education, and an extensive dictionary. The Web site is available in Spanish, but has no support group links.

www.genome.gov

This is the Web site of the National Human Genome Research Institute, National Institutes of Health. The site provides up-to-date status reports on the Human Genome Project, educational resources, a talking glossary, genetics frequently asked questions, and extensive information on careers, training, and grant opportunities in genetics. A sublink is devoted to policy, privacy, and discrimination resources and information. The site does not include a chat room, is only offered in English, and is intended primarily for professionals.

www.ornl.gov/TechResources/Human_Genome/home.html

This Web site is the information source for the Human Genome Project with ongoing and emerging research areas, up-to-date and extensive information on the science of genes, genetic testing, descriptions of genetic diseases and considerations in/for genetic consultation/testing decisions, training/education in genetics, and related medical, ethical, legal, and social issues. The site is informative and useful for both consumers and practitioners. Links are available to locate genetic clinics, counseling and testing services, a directory of genetic support groups, and a glossary of terms in print and "talking" form. The site is offered only in English.

SPECIFICALLY FOR SOCIAL WORKERS

www.aascipsw.org

This Web site is sponsored by the American Association of Spinal Cord Injury Psychologists and Social Workers. The home page has links and information for psychologists and social workers on paper and poster presentations, conferences, abstracts on spinal cord medicine, professional publications and presentations, advocate's toolkit, an annual awards program, and membership. The information provided is directed only toward professionals in the fields of psychology and social work. There are no chat rooms or support groups, glossary, or listing of local providers. The information is provided in English only.

www.nasw.dc.org

The NASW sponsors this Web site supplying information on current social work issues, the organization, membership, publications, professional development, a pressroom, advocacy, resources, a social worker directory, a job link, an NASW merchandise link, a credentialing center, a link for the NASW Foundation and PACE, and a link for a legal defense fund. The site offers a search engine for locating social workers. The Web site is geared toward social work professionals; much of the information is limited to members of the NASW. The Web site does not have chat rooms or support groups, is in English only, and provides no glossary of terms.

ASSESSMENT/MEASUREMENT TOOLS
AND INSTRUMENTS

www.sf-36.org/wantsf.aspx?id=1

This Web site is the licensing and registration site for the SF-36, SF-12, SF-8, and SF-36+Social Work; copyrights are coheld by the Medical Outcomes Trust, Health Assessment Lab and QualityMetric Incorporated. The site offers licensing, measurement scale purchase, online scoring capability, and manuals and video training materials for using each of the measurement scales.

www.walmyr.com/scales.html

This is the Web site of the WALMYR Publishing Company, the publisher of the Hudson Short-Form Assessment Scales, as well as others. The forms are available through the site in paper and computer formats, as are training and scoring manuals for the scales, and reliability and validity statistics are included. All the scales are available by downloading, and can be ordered online, but copyright issues pertain. Costs are generally in the $20 range for pads of multiple scales. Scales include, for example, Brief Adult Assessment Scale, Clinical Anxiety Scale, and Generalized Contentment Scale.

www.health.org/govpubs/BKD250?26k.aspx

This Web site is sponsored by the National Center of Alcohol and Drug Information (NCADI) of the Substance Abuse and Mental Health Services Administration, U.S. Department of Health and Human Services. The NCADI Web site offers several validated and reliable instruments online, including the Alcohol Use Disorders Identification Test (AUDIT), the Index of Activities of Daily Living (ADLs), the Instrumental Activities of Daily Living (IADLs) Scale, and the Geriatric Depression Scale (GDS)– Short Form.

Scoring for each scale is included. The site is intended for professionals; it does not include links for consumers and is offered only in English.

Appendix C

Culturally Related Assessment Topics and Questions

SPIRITUAL ORIENTATION

What beliefs does the consumer/family have concerning higher powers and their own and higher powers' roles in health/illness concerns?
Are prayer/religious practices used? If so, are they used for health concerns?
Is the consumer/family connected to a church, mosque, or temple?
If so, what is its role in the consumer's and/or family's life?
Should members or leaders of the faith organization be included in work with the consumer and family?

HEALTH BELIEFS

What beliefs does the consumer/family have concerning the medical condition and its cause, treatment for the medical condition, and Western biomedicine?
Are ethnocultural health care practices or healers used at all? Currently?
If so, are there conflicts between those and the care and treatment by allopathic practitioners?

FAMILY STRUCTURE, AUTHORITY, AND ROLES

Whom does the consumer and family consider in the family?
Who in the family is/are considered decision makers, particularly for health concerns of family members?
Should these authority figures be included in interviews?
Whom, if anyone, does the consumer prefer to be included in interviews?

Social Work Practice in Community-Based Health Care
© 2007 by The Haworth Press, Inc. All rights reserved.
doi:10.1300/5273_10

If so, are they present and/or to be included in interviews with the social worker and appointments with physicians or other health care providers?
Is anyone the informally designated caregiver for ill family members?

ACCULTURATION

What languages do the consumer and family prefer?
Is an interpreter appropriate?
Are the consumer and/or family members recent immigrants to the United States?
If so, what prompted immigration? Are there presently immigration legalities?
Do the consumer and/or family members have local connections to a community of their cultural background?
To what extent are the consumer and family acculturated to the Western model of biomedicine?

SOCIAL RULES AND VALUES

Does the consumer's family have values or preferences as to the following:
  Who is to be spoken to first? With formal titles?
  Are children to be spoken to directly?
  Possible nonverbal behaviors (i.e., gestures, eye contact, physical proximity)?
  Punctuality and time reference (i.e., clock time and future or present)?
  Length of the session?
Does the consumer's cultural background include beliefs about the consumer's medical condition or disease? If so, are these stigmatizing?

References

Chapter 1

Amonkar, M., Madhavan, S., Rosenbluth, S., Odedina, F., & Simon, K. (2000). Assessing managed care's role in promoting preventive care. *Journal of Community Health, 25*(3), 225-240.

Berkman, B. (1996). The emerging health care world: Implications for practice and education. *Social Work, 41*(5), 541-551.

Berkman, B. & Maramaldi, P. (2001). Use of standardized measures in agency based research and practice. *Social Work in Health Care, 34*(1/2), 115-129.

Boo, M. (1991). *House of stone: The Duluth Benedictines.* Duluth, MN: Scholastica Priory Books.

Calloway, S. & Venegas, L. (2002). The new HIPAA law on privacy and confidentiality. *Nursing Administration, 26*(4), 40-54.

Caputi, M. & Heiss, W. (1984). The DRG revolution. *Health & Social Work, 9*(1), 5-12.

Centers for Medicaid and Medicare Services (2001). *National summary of Medicaid managed care programs and enrollment.* Retrieved April 26, 2004, from www.cms.dhhs.gov/medicaid/managed care/mmcss01.asp.

Centers for Medicaid and Medicare Services (2003). *Projections for 2003.* Retrieved November 11, 2004, from www.cms.hhs.gov/statistics/nhe/projections-2003/proj2003.pdg.

Chambre, S. (2001). The changing nature of "faith" in faith-based organizations: Secularization and ecumenism in four AIDS organizations in New York City. *Social Service Review, 75*(3), 435-455.

Clemmitt, M. (2001). Burgeoning technology will strain Medicare more than previously admitted, says panel. *Medicine & Health Supplement,* February 5, 2-4.

Cnaan, R. & Boddie, S. (2002). Charitable choice and faith-based welfare: A call for social work. *Social Work, 47*(3), 224-245.

Cowles, L. (2003). *Social work in the health field: A care perspective* (2nd ed.). Binghamton, NY: Haworth Press.

Davidson, T., Davidson, J., & Keigher, S. (1999). Managed care: Satisfaction guaranteed . . . Not! *Health & Social Work, 24*(3), 163-171.

Deal, L. & Shiono, P. (1998). Managed care and children: An overview. *The-Future-of-Children, 8*(2), 93-104.

Dinerman, M. (1997). Social work roles in America's changing health care. *Social Work in Health Care, 25*(1/2), 23-33.

Dziegielewski, S. (1998). *The changing face of health care social work: Professional practice in the era of managed care.* New York: Springer Publishing.

Dziegielewski, S. & Holliman, D. (2001). Managed care and social work practice: Implications in an era of change. *Journal of Sociology and Social Welfare, 28*(2), 125-139.

Feldman, R. (2001). Health care and social work education in a changing world. *Social Work in Health Care, 34*(1/2), 31-41.

Friedman, E. (1996). Capitation, integration and managed care. *Journal of the American Medical Association, 275*(12), 957-969.

Gelman, R., Pollack, D., & Weiner, A. (1999). Confidentiality of social work records in the computer age. *Social Work, 44*(3), 243-252.

Gorin, S. (2003). The unraveling of managed care: Recent trends and implications. *Health & Social Work, 28*(3), 241-246.

Hodge, D. & Pittman, J. (2003). Faith-based drug and alcohol treatment providers: An exploratory study of Texan providers. *Journal of Social Service Research, 30*(1), 19-40.

Jensen, G. & Morrisey, M. (2004). Are healthier older adults choosing managed care? *The Gerontologist, 44*(1), 85-94.

Jensen, G., Morrisey, M., Gaffney, S., & Liston, D. (1997). The new dominance of managed care: Insurance trends in the 1990s. *Health Affairs, 6*(1), 125-136.

Kane, M., Houston-Vega, M., & Nuehring, E. (2002). Documentation in managed care: Challenges for social work education. *Journal of Teaching in Social Work, 22*(1/2), 199-212.

Lesser, J. (2000). Clinical social work and family medicine: A partnership in community service. *Health & Social Work, 25*(2), 119-126.

Lowenberg, F., Dolgoff, R., & Harrington, D. (2000). *Ethical decisions for social work practice* (6th ed.). Itasca, IL: Peacock Publishers, Inc.

National Association of Social Workers (NASW) (2001). *Revisions to the NASW code of ethics.* Retrieved May 12, 2005, from www.naswdc.org/pubs/code/code.asp.

Pear, R. (1999). Poor workers lose Medicaid coverage despite eligibility. *New York Times,* April 12, p. 1.

Pecukonis, E., Cornelius, L., & Parrish, M. (2003). The future of health social work. *Social Work in Health Care, 37*(3), 1-15.

Powell, J., Dosser, D., Handron, D., McCammon, S., Temkin, M., & Kaufman, M. (1999). Challenges in interdisciplinary collaboration: A faculty consortium's initial attempts to model collaborative practice. *Journal of Community Practice, 6*(2), 27-48.

Reamer, F. (1997). Managing ethics under managed care. *Families in Society, 78*(1), 96-101.

Redmond, H. (2001). The health care crisis in the United States: A call to action. *Health & Social Work, 26*(1), 54-57.

Rock, B. & Congress, E. (1999). The new confidentiality for the 21st century in a managed care environment. *Social Work, 44*(3), 253-262.

Rosenberg, Gary. (1998). Social work in a health and managed care environment. In G. Schamess, & A. Lightburn (Eds.), *Humane managed care?* (pp. 3-22). Washington, DC: NASW Press.

Schneider, A., Hyer, K., & Luptak, M. (2000). Suggestions to social workers for surviving in managed care. *Health & Social Work, 25*(4), 276-279.

Shadid, M. (1959). *Crusading doctor: My fight for cooperative medicine.* Boston, MA: Meador Publishing Company.

Shortell, S., Gillies, R., & Devers, K. (1995). Reinventing the American hospital. *The Milbank Quarterly, 73*(2), 131-160.

Shortell, S. & Hull, K. (1996). The new organization of the health care delivery system. *Baxter Health Policy Review, 2,* 101-148.

Sherman, A. (2000). Tracking charitable choice: A study of the collaborations between faith-based organizations and the government in providing social services in the United States. *Social Work and Christianity, 27*(2), 112-129.

Starr, P. (1982). *The social transformation of American medicine.* New York: Basic Books.

Starr, P. (1994). *The logic of health care reform: Why and how the president's plan will work.* New York: Whittle/Penguin Books.

Strunk, B., & Ginsburg, B. (2004). Trends: Tracking health care costs: Trends turn downward in 2003 [Web exclusive]. *Health Affairs,* w354-362.

U.S. Department of Health and Human Services, Administration for Children and Families (1999). *Going local: Patch and neighborhood approaches: A transfer from the United Kingdom.* Retrieved December 29, 2004, from www.acf.dhhs.gov/programs/patch.htm.

Volland, P., Berkman, B., Phillips, M., & Stein, G. (2003). Social work education in health care: Addressing practice competencies. *Social Work in Health Care, 37*(4), 1-17.

Weissman, J., Witzburg, R., Linov, P., & Campbell, E. (1999). Termination from Medicaid: How does it affect access, continuity of care, and willingness to purchase insurance? *Journal of Health Care for the Poor and Underserved, 10*(1), 122-147.

The White House (2003). *Faith-based and community initiative.* Retrieved October 29, 2003, from www.whitehouse.gov/government/fbci/html.

Zayas, L. & Dyche, L. (1992). Social workers training primary care physicians: Essential psychosocial principles. *Social Work, 37*(3), 247-252.

Chapter 2

ABC NEWS. (2002). *Number of uninsured up 2 years in a row.* Retrieved October 27, 2003, from http://abcnews.com.

Akinbami, L. & Schoendorf, K. (2002). Trends in childhood asthma: Prevalence, health care utilization, and mortality. *Pediatrics, 110*(2), 315-322.

American Diabetes Association (2005). *Diabetes statistics.* Retrieved May 24, 2005, from www.diabetes.org/diabetes-statistics.

American Lung Association, Epidemiology and Statistics Unit (2003). *Trends in asthma morbidity and mortality.* New York: American Lung Association.

American Heart Association, Epidemiology and Statistics Unit (2004). *Statistical fact sheet—Populations.* Retrieved February 23, 2005, from www.americanheart.org/presenter.jhtml?identifier=2011.

Appel, S., Harrell, J., & Deng, S. (2002). Racial and socioeconomic differences in risk factors for cardiovascular disease among southern rural women. *Nursing Research, 51*(3), 140-147.

Auslander, W., Haire-Joshu, D., Houston, C., Rhee, C-W., & Williams, J. (2002). A controlled evaluation of staging dietary patterns to reduce the risk of diabetes in African-American women. *Diabetes Care, 25*(5), 809-814.

Bennett, T. & Kotelchuck, M. (1997). Mothers and infants. In J. Kotch (Ed.), *Maternal and child health: Programs, problems and policy in public health* (pp. 85-114). Gaithersburg, MD: Aspen.

Berger, C. (2001). Infant mortality: A reflection of the quality of health. *Health & Social Work, 26*(4), 276-282.

Berkman, B., Shearer, S., Simmons, W., White, M., Robinson, M., Sampson, S., et al. (1996). Ambulatory elderly patients of primary care physicians: Functional, psychosocial and environmental predictors of need for social work management. *Social Work in Health Care, 22*(3), 1-21.

Bertera, E. (2003). Psychosocial factors and ethnic disparities in diabetes diagnosis and treatment among older adults. *Health & Social Work, 28*(1), 33-42.

Bontempi, J., Burleson, L., & Lopez, M. (2004). HIV medication adherence programs: The importance of social support. *Journal of Community Health Nursing, 21*(2), 111-122.

Boyd-Franklin, N. (2003). *Black families in therapy: Understanding the African American experience* (2nd ed.). New York: Guilford Press.

Centers for Disease Control (1998). *Summary health stats for U.S.* Retrieved September 14, 2004, from www.cdc.gov.

Centers for Disease Control, Office of Minority Health (2002a). *Eliminating racial and ethnic health disparities.* Retrieved February 23, 2005, from www.cdc.gov/omh/aboutus/disparities.

Centers for Disease Control, National Center for Health Statistics (2002b). *Health: United States.* Retrieved February 23, 2005, from www.cdc.gov/nchs/data/hos/hos04trend.pdf.

Centers for Disease Control, Divisions of HIV, STD and TB Prevention, National Center for HIV/STD and TB (2003a). *HIV/AIDS Surveillance Supplemental Report, 10*(1). Retrieved September 8, 2004, from www.cdc.gov/his/stats/hasrsupp10.1htm.

Centers for Disease Control, Office of Disease Prevention and Health Promotion (2003b). *Fact sheet: Healthy people 2010.* Atlanta, GA: Centers for Disease Control. Retrieved February 22, 2004, from www.cdc.gov/diabetes/pubs/pdf/ndfs-2003.pdf.

Clark, N., Brown, R., Joseph, C., Anderson, E., Liu, M., & Valerio, M. (2004). Effects of a comprehensive school-based asthma program on symptoms, parent management, grades and absenteeism. *Chest, 125*(5), 1674-1679.

CNN News (March 17, 2004). *Hispanic, Asian populations to triple by 2050.* Retrieved March 24, 2004, from www.cnn.usnews.com.

Cornelius, D. (2000). Financial barriers to health care for Latinos: Poverty and beyond. *Journal of Poverty, 4*(1/2), 63-83.

Crespo, C. & Arbesman, J. (2003). Obesity in the United States. *Physician and Sports Medicine, 31*(11), 23-29.

Cunningham, M. & Zayas, L. (2002). Reducing depression in pregnancy: Designing multimodal interventions. *Social Work, 47*(2), 114-124.

DeCoster, V. (2003). The emotions of adults with diabetes: A comparison across race. *Social Work in Health Care, 36*(4), 79-99.

DeCoster, V. & Cummings, S. (2004). Coping with type 2 diabetes: Do race and gender matter? *Social Work in Health Care, 40*(2), 37-53.

Degeneffe, C. (2001). Family caregiving and traumatic brain injury. *Health & Social Work, 26*(4), 257-268.

Dhooper, S. (2003). Health care needs of foreign-born Asian Americans: An overview. *Health & Social Work, 28*(1), 63-73.

Diabetes Week. Editors (2004). *Study shows diabetes disease management reduces costs, improves quality.* Retrieved September, 21, 2004, from www.NewsRx.com.

Donelan, K., Blendon, R., Hill, C., Hoffman, C., Rowland, C., Frankel, M., et al. (1996). Whatever happened to the health insurance crisis in the United States: Voices from a national survey. *Journal of the American Medical Association, 276,* 1346-1350.

Flegal, K., Carroll, M., Ogden, C., & Johnson, C. (2002). Prevalence and trends in obesity among U.S. adults, 1999-2000. *Journal of the American Medical Association, 288*(14), 1723-1727.

Galambos, C. (2003). Moving cultural diversity toward cultural competence in health care. *Health & Social Work, 28*(1), 3-6.

Gorin, S. & Moniz, C. (2004). Will the United States ever have universal health care? *Health & Social Work, 29*(4), 340-344.

Hafner-Eaton, C. (1994). Patterns of hospital and physician utilization among the uninsured. *Journal of the Poor and Underserved, 5*(4), 297-315.

Harris, M. & Franklin, C. (2003). Effects of a cognitive-behavioral, school-based, group intervention with Mexican American pregnant and parenting adolescents. *Social Work Research, 27*(2), 71-83.

Hobbs, F. & Damon, B. (1996). *65+ in the United States.* Retrieved August 15, 2003, from www.census.gov/prod/1/pop/html.

Institute of Medicine (IOM) (2001). *Health behavior: The interplay between biological, behavioral, and societal influences.* Washington, DC: National Academy Press.

Institute of Medicine (IOM) (2002). *Unequal treatment: Confronting racial and ethnic disparities in health care.* Retrieved Sept. 8, 2004, from www.iom.edu/report.

Kaiser Commission on Medicaid and the Uninsured (2004). *Uninsured in America: A chart book.* Washington, DC: The Kaiser Family Foundation.

Kaiser Family Foundation (2004). *Racial and ethnic disparities in women's health coverage and access to care: Findings from the 2001 Kaiser Women's Health Survey.* Washington, DC: Author.

Keigher, S. (1997). What role for social work in the new health care practice paradigm? *Health & Social Work, 22*(2), 149-155.

Logsdon, M. & Davis, D. (2003). Social and professional support for pregnant and parenting women. *The American Journal of Maternal-Child Nursing, 28*(6), 371-376.

Maljanian, R., Grey, N., Staff, I., & Cruz-Marino-Aponte, M. (2002). Improved diabetes control through a provider-based disease management program. *Disease Managed Health Outcomes, 10*(1), 1-8.

Mason, J., Edlow, M., Lear, M., Scoppetta, S., Walther, V., Epstein, I., et al. (2001). Screening for psychosocial risk in an urban prenatal clinic: A retrospective practice-based research study. *Social Work in Health Care, 33*(3/4), 33-52.

Mitchell, C. & Linsk, M. (2004). A multidimensional conceptual framework for understanding HIV/AIDS as a chronic long-term illness. *Social Work, 49*(3), 469-477.

National Rural Health Association (NRHA) (2003). *Access to health care for the uninsured in rural and frontier America.* Retrieved December 5, 2003, from www.nrharural.org/pagefileissuepapersipaper15.html.

Navaie-Waliser, M., Martin, S., Tessaro, I., Campbell, M., & Cross, A. (2000). Social support and psychological functioning among high risk mothers: The impact of the Baby Love Maternal Outreach Worker Program. *Public Health Nursing, 17*, 280-291.

Pecukonis, E., Cornelius, L., & Parrish, M. (2003). The future of health social work. *Social Work in Health Care, 37*(3), 1-15.

Philis-Tsimikas, A. & Walker, C. (2001). Improved care for diabetes in underserved populations. *Journal of Ambulatory Care, 24*(1), 39-43.

Pinquart, M. & Sorensen, S. (2005). Ethnic differences in stressors, resources, and psychological outcomes of family caregiving: A meta-analysis. *The Gerontologist, 45*, 90-106.

Polonsky, W., Earles, J., Smith, S., Pease, D., Macmillan, M., Christensen, R., et al. (2003). Integrating medical management with diabetes self-management training. *Diabetes Care, 26*(11), 3048-3053.

Rivera, P., Shewchuk, R., & Elliott, T. (2003). Project FOCUS: Using videophones to provide problem-solving training to family caregivers of persons with spinal cord injuries. *Spinal Cord Injury Rehabilitation, 9*(1), 53-62.

Sharma, R. (1998). Causal pathways to infant mortality: Linking social variables to infant mortality through intermediate variables. *Journal of Health and Social Policy, 9*(3), 15-28.

Sudha, S. & Multran, E. (2001). Race, ethnicity, nativity, and issues of health. *Research on Aging, 23*(1), 3-13.

Thompson, S., Auslander, W., & White, N. (2001). Influence of family structure on health among youths with diabetes. *Health & Social Work, 26*(1), 7-14.

Tinkelman, D. & Schwartz, A. (2004). School-based asthma disease management. *Journal of Asthma, 41*(4), 455-462.

U.S. Census Bureau (1998). *Report on the uninsured in America.* Retrieved July 18, 2004, from www.cdc.gov/nchs.

U.S. Census Bureau (2000a). *Projected life expectancy at birth by race and Hispanic origin, 1999-2100.* Retrieved July 18, 2004, from www.cdc.gov/nchs.

U.S. Census Bureau (2000b). *Population projections program.* Retrieved July 18, 2004, from www.census.gov/nchs.

U.S. Census Bureau (2003). *Income, poverty, and health insurance coverage in the United States.* Retrieved October 17, 2004, from www.cdc.gov/nchs.

U.S. Census Bureau (2004). *Health insurance coverage.* Retrieved October 17, 2004, from www.census.gov/prod/2004pubs/p60-226.pdf.

U.S. Department of Health and Human Services (2001). *Diabetes fact sheet.* Retrieved September 21, 2004, from www.ahrq.gov.

U.S. Department of Health and Human Services (2002). *Healthy people 2010 fact sheet.* Washington, DC: DHHS. Retrieved September 8, 2004, from www.healthypeople.gov.

U.S. Office of Women's Health (2004). *The health of minority women. Barriers limiting access to health care.* Retrieved September 27, 2004, from www.4women.gov.

Van Loon, R., Borkin, R., & Steffen, J. (2002). Health care experiences and preferences of uninsured workers. *Health & Social Work, 27*(1), 17-26.

Volland, P., Berkman, B., Phillips, M., & Stein, G. (2003). Social work education for health care: Addressing practice competencies. *Social Work in Health Care, 37*(4), 1-17.

Vourlekis, B., Ell, K., & Padgett, D. (2001). Educating social workers for health care's brave new world. *Journal of Social Work Education, 37*(1), 177-191.

Webber, M., Carpiniello, K., Oruwariye, T., Lo, Y., Burton, W., & Appel, D. (2003). Burden of asthma in inner-city elementary schoolchildren: Do school-based health centers make a difference? *Archives of Pediatric Adolescent Medicine, 157*, 125-129.

Weissman, J., Witzburg, R., Linov, P., & Campbell, E. (1999). Termination from Medicaid: How does it affect access, continuity of care, and willingness to purchase insurance? *Journal of Health Care for the Poor and Underserved, 10*(1), 122-147.

Widerman, E. (2004). The experience of receiving a diagnosis of Cystic Fibrosis after the age of 20: Implications for social work. *Social Work in Health Care, 39*(3/4), 415-433.

Willoughby, D., Kee, C., & Demi, A. (2000). Women's psychosocial adjustment to diabetes. *Journal of Advanced Nursing, 32,* 1422-1430.

Zebrack, B. & Chesler, M. (2000). Managed care: The new context for social work in health care: Implications for survivors of childhood cancer and their families. *Social Work in Health Care, 31*(2), 89-103.

Zebrack, B. & Chesler, M. (2001). Health-related worries, self-image and life outlooks of long-term survivors of childhood cancer. *Health & Social Work, 26*(4), 245-256.

Chapter 3

Al-Krenawi, A. & Graham, J. (2000a). Culturally sensitive social work practice with Arab clients in mental health settings. *Health & Social Work, 25*(1), 9-22.

Al-Krenawi, A. & Graham, J. (2000b). Islamic theology and prayer: Relevance for social work practice. *International Social Work, 43*(3), 289-304.

Appel, S., Harrell, J., & Deng, S. (2002). Racial and socioeconomic differences in risk factors for cardiovascular disease among southern rural women. *Nursing Research, 51*(3), 140-147.

Applewhite, S. (1995). *Curanderismo:* Demystifying the health beliefs and practices of elderly Mexican Americans. *Health & Social Work, 20,* 247-253.

Aranda, M. & Knight, B. (1997). The influence of ethnicity and culture on the caregiver stress and coping process: A sociocultural review and analysis. *The Gerontologist, 17*(3), 342-354.

Barnes, S. (2001). Stressors and strengths: A theoretical and practical examination of nuclear, single-parent, and augmented African American families. *Families in Society, 82*(5), 449-460.

Barrios, T. & Egan, M. (2002). Living in a bi-cultural world and finding the way home: Native women's stories. *Affilia: Journal of Women and Social Work, 17*(2), 206-228.

Billingsley, A. (1999). *Mighty like a river: The black church and social reform.* New York: Oxford University Press.

Blackhall, L., Frank, G., Murphy, S., Michel, V., Palmer, J., & Azen, S. (1999). Ethnicity and attitudes towards life sustaining technology. *Social Science & Medicine, 48,* 1779-1789.

Boyd-Franklin, N. (2003). *Black families in therapy: Understanding the African American experience* (2nd ed.). New York: Guilford Press.

Brach, C. & Fraser, I. (2000). Can cultural competency reduce racial and ethnic health disparities? A review and conceptual model. *Medical Care Research and Review, 57,* 181-217.

Campinha-Bacote, J. (2002). The process of cultural competence in the delivery of healthcare services: A model of care. *Journal of Transcultural Nursing, 13*(3), 182-184.

Chadiha, L., Proctor, E., Morrow-Howell, N., Darkwa, O., & Dore, P. (1996). Religiosity and church-based assistance among chronically ill African-American and White elderly. *Journal of Religious Gerontology, 10*(1), 17-36.

Chin, J. (2000). Culturally competent health care. *Public Health Reports, 115*(1), 25-38.

Chillag, K., Bartholow, K., Cordeiro, J., Swanson, S., Patterson, J., Stebbins, S., et al. (2002). Factors affecting the delivery of HIV/AIDS prevention programs by community-based organizations. *AIDS Education and Prevention, 14*(3/ Supp.), 27-37.

Congress, E. (2004). Cultural and ethical issues in working with culturally diverse patients and their families: The use of the Culturagram to promote cultural competent practice in health care settings. *Social Work in Health Care, 39*(3/4), 249-262.

DeCoster, V. & Cummings, S. (2004). Coping with type 2 diabetes: Do race and gender matter? *Social Work in Health Care, 40*(2), 37-53.

Dhooper, S. (2003). Health care needs of foreign-born Asian Americans: An overview. *Health & Social Work, 28*(1), 63-73.

Dhooper, S. & Tran, T. (1998). Understanding and responding to the health and mental health needs of Asian refugees. *Social Work in Health Care, 27*(4), 65-82.

Dosser, D., Smith, A., Markowski, E., & Cain, H. (2001). Including families' spiritual beliefs and their faith communities in systems of care. *Journal of Family Social Work, 5*(3), 63-78.

Galan, F. (2001). Experiential approach with Mexican-American males with acculturation stress. In H. Briggs, & K. Corcoran (Eds.), *Social work practice: Treating common client problems* (pp. 283-302). Chicago, IL: Lyceum Books, Inc.

Green, J. (1999). *Cultural awareness in the human services: A multi-ethnic approach* (3rd ed.). Needham, MA: Allyn & Bacon.

Gorin, S. (2001). The crisis of public health: Implications for social workers. *Health & Social Work, 26*(1), 49-53.

Hodge, D. (2004). Working with Hindu clients in a spiritually sensitive manner. *Social Work, 49*(1), 27-38.

Imes, S. & Landry, D. (2002). Don't underestimate the power of culture. *Science of Nursing, 19*(4), 172-176.

Institute of Medicine (2002). *Unequal treatment: Confronting racial and ethnic disparities in health care.* Retrieved June 15, 2004, from http://www.iom.edu/iomhome.

Jackson, L. (1993). Understanding, eliciting, and negotiating clients' multicultural health beliefs. *Nurse Practitioner, 18*(4), 30-43.

Kemper, K. & Barnes, L. (2003). Considering culture, complementary medicine, and spirituality in pediatrics. *Clinical Pediatrics, 42,* 205-208.

LaViest, T. (1994). Beyond dummy variables and sample selection: What health services researchers ought to know about race as a variable. *Health Services Research, 29,* 1-17.

Leininger, M. (1991). *Cultural care diversity and universality: A theory of nursing.* New York: National League for Nursing Press.

Lum, Y., Chang, H., & Ozawa, M. (1999). The effects of race and ethnicity on use of health services by older Americans. *Journal of Social Service Research, 25*(4), 15-42.

Luna, I., de Ardon, E., Lim, Y., Cromwell, S., Phillips, L., & Russel, C. (1996). Relevance of familism in cross-cultural studies in family caregiving. *Western Journal of Nursing Research, 18*(3), 267-283.

Ma, G. (1999). Between two worlds: The use of traditional and Western health services by Chinese Americans. *Journal of Community Health, 24*(6), 421-437.

McCullough, M., Hoyt, W. Larson, D. Koenig, H., & Thoreson, C. (2000). Religious involvement and mortality: A meta-analytic review. *Health Psychology, 19*(3), 211-222.

McEvoy, M. (2003). Culture and spirituality as an integrated concept in pediatric care. *American Journal of Maternal Child Nursing, 28*(1), 39-44.

Murguia, A., Peterson, R., & Zea, M. (2003). Use and implications of ethnomedical health care approaches among Central American Immigrants. *Health & Social Work, 28*(1), 43-52.

Murguia, A., Zea, M., Reisen, C., & Peterson, R. (2000). The development of the Cultural Attributions Questionnaire (CHAQ). *Cultural Diversity and Ethnic Minority Physicians, 6*(3), 258-283.

Murphy, J. (1993). *Santeria: African spirits in America.* Boston, MA: Beacon Press.

National Association of Social Workers (NASW). (June 23, 2001). *Standards for cultural competence in social work practice.* Retrieved, June 9, 2005, from www.socialworkers.org/sections/credentials/cultural_comp.asp.

National Center for Complementary and Alternative Medicine (2002). *What is complementary and alternative medicine (CAM).* Retrieved April 5, 2005, from www.nccam.nih.gov/health/whatiscam.

National Center for Complementary and Alternative Medicine (2004). *The use of complementary and alternative medicine in the United States, 2002.* Retrieved April 5, 2005, from www.nccam.nih.gov/news/camsurvey_fs.htm.

National Institutes of Health (NIH) (2004). *CDC Advance Data Report #343: Complementary and alternative medicine use among adults: United States, 2002.* Retrieved April 5, 2005, from www.nih.gov.news/camsurvey.htm.

Nobles, A. & Sciarra, D. (2000). Cultural determinants in the treatment of Arab Americans: A primer for mainstream therapists. *Journal of Orthopsychiatry, 20*(2), 182-191.

Nunez, A. (2000). Transforming cultural competence into cross-cultural efficacy in women's health education. *Academic Medicine, 75,* 1071-1080.

Ow, R. & Katz, D. (1999). Family secrets and the disclosure of distressful information in Chinese families. *Families in Society, 80*(6), 620-628.

Pachter, L. (1994). Culture and clinical care. *Journal of the American Medical Association, 271*(9), 690-712.

Pachter, L., Cloutier, M., & Bernstein, B. (1995). Ethnomedical (folk) remedies for childhood asthma in a mainland Puerto Rican community. *Archives of Pediatric Adolescent Medicine, 149,* 982-988.

Panos, P. & Panos, A. (2000). A model for a culture-sensitive assessment of patients in health care settings. *Social Work in Health Care, 31*(1), 49-62.

Porter, E., Gnong, L., & Armer, J. (2000). The church family and kin: An older rural black woman's support network and preferences for care provider. *Qualitative Health Research, 10*(4), 452-470.

Schilder, A., Kennedy, C., Goldstone, I., Ogden, R., Hogg, & O'Shaugnessy, M. (2001). "Being dealt with as a whole person." Care seeking and adherence: The benefits of culturally competent care. *Social Science & Medicine, 52,* 1643-1659.

Sudha, S. & Multran, E. (2001). Race and ethnicity, nativity, and issues of health care. *Research on Aging, 23*(1), 3-13.

Thobaben, M. (2002). Racial and ethnic disparities in health care. *Community-Based Health Care Management and Practice, 14*(6), 479-481.

U.S. Department of Health and Human Services, Public Health Service, Office of Minority Health (2001). *National standards for culturally and linguistically ap-*

propriate service in health care: Final report. Retrieved September 14, 2003, from http://www.omhrc.gov/clas/index/htm.

U.S. Department of Health and Human Services (2002). *Healthy people 2010 fact sheet.* Retrieved Sept. 8, 2004, from www.healthypeople.gov/About/hpfact.htm.

Van Hook, M., Hugen, B., & Aguilar, M. (2001). *Spirituality within religious traditions in social work practice.* Pacific Grove, CA: Brooks/Cole.

Van Loon, R., Borkin, R., & Steffen, J. (2002). Health care experiences and preferences of uninsured workers. *Health & Social Work, 27*(1), 17-26.

Voss, R., Douville, V., Soldier, A., & Twiss, G. (1999). Tribal and shamanic-based social work practice: A Lakota perspective. *Social Work, 44*(3), 228-241.

Walters, K. (1999). Urban American Indian identity attitudes and acculturation styles. *Journal of Human Behavior in the Social Environment, 2*(1/2), 163-178.

Weaver, H. (2003). *Voices of first nations people.* Binghamton, NY: Haworth Press.

Weaver, H. (2005). *Explorations in cultural competence: Journeys to the four directions.* Belmont, CA: Thomson/Brooks/Cole.

Weaver, H. & White, B. (1997). The Native American family circle: Roots of resiliency. *Journal of Family Social Work, 2*(1), 67-79.

White, T., Townsend, A., & Stephens, M. (2000). Comparisons of African American and white women in the parent care role. *The Gerontologist, 40*(6), 718-728.

Williams, S. & Dilworth-Anderson, P. (2002). Systems of social support in families who care for dependent African American elders. *The Gerontologist, 42*(2), 224-236.

Zayas, L. & Dyche, L. (1992). Social workers training primary care physicians: Essential psychosocial principles. *Social Work, 37*(3), 247-252.

Chapter 4

Auslander, W., Haire-Joshu, D., Houston, C., Rhee, C-W., & Williams, J. (2002). A controlled evaluation of staging dietary patterns to reduce the risk of diabetes in African American women. *Diabetes Care, 25*(5), 809-814.

Badger, L., Ackerson, B., Buttell, J., & Rand, E. (1997). The case for integration of social work psychological services into rural primary care. *Health & Social Work, 22*(1), 20-29.

Berkman, B., Shearer, S., Simmons, W., White, M., Robinson, M., Sampson, S., et al. (1996). Ambulatory elderly patients of primary care physicians: Functional, psychosocial and environmental predictors of need for social work management. *Social Work in Health Care, 22*(3), 1-21.

Bindman, A., Grumbach, K., Osmond, D., Vranizan, K., & Stewart, A. (1996). Primary care and receipt of preventive services. *Journal of General Internal Medicine, 11*(5), 269-276.

Brook, D., Gordon, C., Meadow, H., & Cohen, M. (2000). Behavioral medicine in medical education: Report of a survey. *Social Work in Health Care, 31*(2), 15-29.

Cameron, J. & Mauksch, L. (2002). Collaborative family health care in an uninsured primary care population: Stages of integration. *Family, Systems and Health, 20,* 343-363.

Claiborne, N. & Vandenburgh, H. (2001). Social workers' role in disease management. *Health & Social Work, 26*(4), 217-225.

Clemmitt, M. (2001). Burgeoning technology will strain Medicare more than previously admitted, says panel. *Medicine & Health Supplement,* February 5, 2-4.

Comer, E. (2004). Integrating the health and mental health needs of the chronically ill: A group of individuals with depression and sickle cell disease. *Social Work in Health Care, 38*(4), 57-76.

Corwin, M. (2002). Brief social work practice in health care. In M. Corwin (Ed.), *Brief treatment in clinical social work practice* (pp. 181-221). Pacific Grove, CA: Brooks/Cole.

Cowles, L. (2003). Social work in primary care settings. In L. Cowles (Ed.), *Social work in the health field: A care perspective* (2nd ed., pp. 87-142). Binghamton, NY: Haworth Press.

DeCoster, V. & Egan, M. (2001). Physicians' perceptions and responses to patient emotion: Implications for social work practice in health care. *Social Work in Health Care, 32*(3), 21-40.

Dziegielewski, S. (2004). *The changing face of health care social work: Professional practice in an era of managed care* (2nd ed.). New York: Springer Publishing.

Dziegielewski, S. & Holliman, D. (2001). Managed care and social work practice: Implications in an era of change. *Journal of Sociology and Social Welfare, 28*(2), 125-139.

Farmer, J. & Muhlenbruck, L. (2001). Telehealth for children with special health care needs: Promoting comprehensive systems of care. *Clinical Pediatrics, 40,* 93-98.

Feldman, R. (2001). Health care and social work education in a changing world. *Social Work, 34*(1/2), 31-41.

Freedman, T. (1998). Genetic susceptibility testing: Ethical and social quandaries. *Health & Social Work, 23*(3), 214-232.

Galambos, C. (2003). Building healthy environments: Community- and consumer-based initiatives. *Health & Social Work, 28*(3), 171-174.

Gibelman, M. (2003). *Navigating human service organizations.* Chicago, IL: Lyceum Books.

Harris, M. & Franklin, C. (2003). Effects of a cognitive-behavioral, school-based, group intervention with Mexican American pregnant and parenting adolescents. *Social Work Research, 27*(2), 71-83.

Heckman, T., Kalichman, S., Roffman, R., Sikkema, L., Heckman, B., Somlai, A., et al. (1999). A telephone-delivered coping improvement intervention for persons living with HIV/AIDS in rural areas. *Social Work with Groups, 21*(4), 49-61.

Hunter, D. & Fairfield, G. (1997). Managed care: Disease management. *British Medical Journal, 315,* July 5, 50-53.

Institute of Medicine (IOM) (1994). *Defining primary care: An interim report.* Washington, DC: National Academy Press.

Institute of Medicine (IOM) (2001). *Health behavior: The interplay between biological, behavioral, and societal influences.* Washington, DC: National Academy Press.

Kao, A., Green, D., Zaslavsky, A., Koplan, J., & Cleary, P. (1998). Patient's trust in their physicians: Effects of choice, continuity, and payment method. *Journal of American Medical Association, 280*(19), 1708-1714.

Lesser, J. (2000). Clinical social work and family medicine: A partnership in community service. *Health & Social Work, 25*(2), 119-126.

Lowenberg, F., Dolgoff, R., & Harrington, D. (2000). *Ethical decisions for social work practice* (6th ed.). Itasca, IL: Peacock Publishers.

Lymbery, M. & Milward, A. (2001). Community care in practice: Social work in primary health care. *Social Work in Health Care, 34*(3/4), 241-259.

Mauksch, L., Tucker, S., Katon, W., Russo, J., Cameron, J., & Walker, E. (2001). Mental illness, functional impairment, and patient preferences for collaborative care in an uninsured, primary care population. *Journal of Family Practice, 50*(1), 41-47.

Mosley, A. (1998). Community partnerships in neighborhood-based health care: A response to diminishing resources. *Health & Social Work, 23*(3), 231-235.

National Association of Social Workers (2001). *The NASW code of ethics.* Retrieved March 29, 2005, from www.naswdc.org/pubs/code.

National Human Genome Research Institute (May 2005). *Specific genetic disorders.* Retrieved June 8, 2005, from www.genome.org.

Netting, F. & Williams, F. (2000). Expanding the boundaries of primary care for elderly people. *Health & Social Work, 25*(4), 233-242.

Oktay, J. (2005). *Breast cancer: Daughters tell their stories.* Binghamton, NY: Haworth Press.

Olfson, M., Shea, S., Feder, A., Fuentes, M., Nomura, Y., Gameroff, M., et al. (2000). Prevalence of anxiety, depression, and substance abuse disorders in an urban general medicine practice. *Archives of Family Medicine, 9,* 876-883.

Petrosky, M., Shaffer, C., Devlin, L., & Almog, D. (2000). On-site social work program in an urban academic dental center. *Journal of Dental Education, 64*(5), 370-372.

Pew Internet and American Life Project (November, 2000). *The online revolution: How the Web helps Americans take better care of themselves.* Retrieved January 22, 2004, from www.pewinternet.org/pdf/PIP_Health_Report.pdf.

Piette, J., Kraemer, F., Weinberger, M., & McPhee, S. (2001). Impact of automated calls with nurse follow-up on diabetes treatment outcomes in a Department of Veterans Affairs health care system. *Diabetes Care, 24*(2), 202-208.

Poole, D. & Van Hook, M. (1997). Retooling for community health partnerships in primary care settings. *Health & Social Work, 22*(1), 1-3.

Rock, B. & Congress, E. (1999). The new confidentiality for the 21st century in a managed care environment. *Social Work, 44,* 253-262.

Rock, B. & Cooper, M. (2000). Social work in primary care: A demonstration student unit utilizing practice research. *Social Work in Health Care, 31*(1), 1-15.

Rosenberg, G. & Holden, G. (1997). The role of social work in improving quality of life in the community. *Social Work in Health Care, 25*(1/2), 9-22.

Rudolph, C. (2000). Educational challenges facing health care social workers in the twenty-first century. *Professional Development, 3*(1), 31-43.

Schilder, A., Kennedy, C., Goldstone, I., Ogden, R., Hogg, R., & O'Shaugnessy, M. (2001). "Being dealt with as a whole person." Care seeking and adherence: The benefits of culturally competent care. *Social Science & Medicine, 52*, 1643-1659.

Scholle, S. & Kelleher, K. (1999). Assessing primary care performance in an obstetrics/gynecology clinic. *Women & Health, 37*(1), 15-30.

Simonian, S. & Tarnowski (2001). Utility of the pediatric symptom checklist for behavioral screening of disadvantaged children. *Child Psychiatry and Human Development, 31*(4), 269-278.

Starr, P. (1982). *The social transformation of American medicine.* New York: Basic Books.

Steinman, K., Steinman, M., & Steinman, T. (2003). Disease management programs in the geriatric setting: Practical considerations. *Disease Management and Health Outcomes, 11*(6), 363-374.

Tinkelman, D. & Schwartz, A. (2004). School-based asthma disease management. *Journal of Asthma, 41*(4), 455-462.

Van Hook, M. (2003). Psychosocial issues within primary health care settings: Challenges and opportunities for social work practice. *Social Work in Health Care, 38*(1), 63-80.

Volland, P. (1996). Social work practice in health care: Looking to the future with a different lens. *Social Work in Health Care, 24*(1/2), 35-51.

Waldrop, D., Fabiano, J., Davis, E., Goldberg, L., & Nochajski, T. (2004). Coexistent concerns: Assessing the social and health needs of dental clinic patients. *Social Work in Health Care, 40*(1), 33-51.

Weiss, L. & Blustein, J. (1996). Faithful patients: The effect of long-term physician-patient relationships on the costs and use of health care by older Americans. *American Journal of Public Health, 86*, 1742-1747.

Chapter 5

Abramson, J. & Mizrahi, T. (2003). Understanding collaboration between social workers and physicians: Application of a typology. *Social Work in Health Care, 37*(2), 71-100.

Alter, C. & Egan, M. (1997). Logic modeling: A tool for teaching critical thinking in social work practice. *Journal of Social Work Education, 33*(1), 85-102.

Amyotrophic Lateral Sclerosis (ALS)Association (2004). *Products/services to aid in daily living: Augmentative communication devices.* Retrieved June 6, 2005, from www.als.org/products.cfin.

Beck, J. (1995). *Cognitive therapy: Basics and beyond.* New York: Guilford Press.

Bentley, K., Walsh, J., & Farmer R. (2005). Referring clients for psychiatric medication: Best practices for social workers. *Best Practices in Mental Health, 1*(1), 59-71.

Berkman, B., Chauncey, S., Holmes, W., Daniels, A., Bonander, E., Sampson, S., et al. (1999). Standardized screening for elderly patients' needs for social work assessment in primary care. *Health & Social Work, 24*(1), 9-16.

Berkman, B. & Maramaldi, P. (2001). Use of standardized measures in agency based research and practice. *Social Work in Health Care, 34*(1/2), 115-129.

Boyd-Franklin, N. (2003). *Black families in therapy: Understanding the African American experience* (2nd ed.). New York: Guilford Press.

Cameron, J. & Mauksch, L. (2002). Collaborative family health care in an uninsured primary care population: Stages of integration. *Family, Systems and Health, 20*, 343-363.

Chernesky, R. & Grube, B. (2000). Examining the HIV/AIDS case management process. *Health & Social Work, 25*(4), 243-254.

Claiborne, N. & Massaro, E. (2000). Mental quality of life: An indicator of unmet needs in patients with diabetes. *Social Work in Health Care, 32*(1), 25-43.

Claiborne, N. & Vandenburgh, H. (2001). Social workers' role in disease management. *Health & Social Work, 26*(4), 217-225.

Comer, E. (2004). Integrating the health and mental health needs of the chronically ill: A group of individuals with depression and sickle cell disease. *Social Work in Health Care, 38*(4), 57-76.

Comer, E., Kramer, K., & Nash, K. (2000). Augmenting traditional health care through mutual assistance groups. In S. Logan, & E. Freeman (Eds.), *Health care in the black community* (pp. 215-228). Binghamton, NY: Haworth Press.

Congress, E. (2000). What social workers should know about ethics: Understanding and resolving practice dilemmas. *Advances in Social Work, 1*(1), 1-22.

Congress, E. (2004). Cultural and ethical issues in working with culturally diverse patients and their families: The use of the Culturagram to promote culturally competent practice in health care settings. *Social Work in Health Care, 39*(3/4), 249-262.

Corwin, M. (2002). *Brief treatment in clinical social work practice*. Pacific Grove, CA: Brooks/Cole.

Cruess, S., Antoni, M., Hayes, A., Penedo, F., Ironson, G., Fletcher, M., et al. (2002). Changes in mood and depressive symptoms and related change processes during cognitive-behavioral stress management in HIV-infected men. *Cognitive Therapy and Research, 26*(3), 373-392.

DeCoster, V. & Egan, M. (2001). Physicians' perceptions and responses to patient emotion: Implications for social work practice in health care. *Social Work in Health Care, 32*(3), 21-40.

Dodd, S.-J. & Jansson, B. (2004). Expanding boundaries of ethics education: Preparing social workers for ethical advocacy in an organizational setting. *Journal of Social Work Education, 40*(3), 455-465.

Dziegielewski, S. & Holliman, D. (2001). Managed care and social work practice: Implications in an era of change. *Journal of Sociology and Social Welfare, 28*(2), 125-139.

Finger, W. & Arnold, E. (2002). Mind-body interventions: Applications for social work practice. *Social Work in Health Care, 35*(4), 57-78.

Flores, G. (2000). The teaching of cultural issues in U.S. and Canadian medical schools. *Journal of the American Medical Association, 284*(3), 284-290.

Franklin, C. & Corcoran, J. (2000). Preventing adolescent pregnancy: A review of programs and practices. *Social Work, 45*, 40-52.

Galinsky, M., Schopler, J., & Abell, M. (1997). Connecting group members through telephone and computer groups. *Health & Social Work, 22*(3), 181-188.

Gambrill, E. (1997). *Social work practice: A critical thinker's guide.* New York: Oxford University Press.

Harris, M. & Franklin, C. (2003). Effects of a cognitive-behavioral school-based, group intervention with Mexican American pregnant and parenting adolescents. *Social Work Research, 27*(2), 71-83.

Heckman, T., Kalichman, S., Hoffman, R., Ikea, L., Heckman, B., Somali, A., et al. (1999). A telephone-delivered coping improvement intervention for persons living with HIV/AIDS in rural areas. *Social Work with Groups, 21*(4), 49-61.

Hepworth, D., Rooney, R., & Larsen, J. (2002). *Direct social work practice: Theory and skills* (6th ed.). Pacific Grove, CA: Brooks/Cole-Thomson Learning.

Hunter, D. & Fairfield, G. (1997). Managed care: Disease management. *British Medical Journal, 315,* July 5, 50-54.

Kane, M., Houston-Vega, M., & Neuring, E. (2002). Documentation in managed care: Challenges for social work education. *Journal of Teaching in Social Work, 22*(1), 199-212.

Lazarus, R. & Folkman, S. (1984). *Stress, appraisal and coping.* New York: Springer Publishing.

Leon, A. & Dziegielewski, S. (2000). Engaging Hispanic immigrant mothers: Revisiting the time-limited psycho-educational group model. *Crisis Intervention, 6*(1), 13-27.

Lesser, J. (2000). Clinical social work and family medicine: A partnership in community service. *Health & Social Work, 25*(2), 119-126.

Ligon, J. (1998). Promoting self-management of chronic medical problems. In J. Wodarski, & B. Thyer (Eds.), *Handbook of empirical social work practice,* Volume 2: *Social problems and practice issues* (pp. 299-313). New York: Wiley and Sons.

Lowenberg, F., Dolgoff, R., & Harrington, D. (2000). *Ethical decisions for social work practice* (6th ed.). Itasca, IL: Peacock Publishers.

Mannix, L., Chandurkar, R., Rybicki, L., Tusek, D., & Solomon, G. (1999). Effect of guided imagery on quality of life of patients with chronic tension-type headaches. *Headaches, 39,* 326-334.

Maramaldi, P., Berkman, B., & Barusch, A. (2005). Assessment and the ubiquity of culture: Threats to validity in measures of health-related quality of life. *Health & Social Work, 30*(1), 27-39.

McCarty, D. & Clancy, C. (2002). Tele-health: Implications for social work practice. *Social Work, 47*(2), 153-161.

Millstein, K. (2000). Confidentiality in direct practice: Inevitable challenges ethical dilemmas. *Families in Society: The Journal of Contemporary Human Services, 81*(3), 270-282.

National Association of Social Workers (2001). *The NASW code of ethics.* Retrieved May 2, 2005, from www.naswdc.org/pubs/code/code.asp.

National Center for Complementary and Alternative Medicine (2002). *What is complementary and alternative medicine (CAM).* Retrieved April 5, 2005, from www.nccam.nih.gov/health/whatiscam.

National Center for Complementary and Alternative Medicine (2004). *The use of complementary and alternative medicine in the United States, 2002.* Retrieved April 5, 2005, from www.nccam.nih.gov/news/camsurvey_fs.htm.

Netting, F. & Williams, F. (2000). Expanding the boundaries of primary care for elderly people. *Health & Social Work, 25*(4), 233-242.

Roffman, R., Picciano, J., Ryan, R., Beadnall, B., Fisher, D., Downey, L., et al. (1997). HIV prevention group counseling delivered by telephone: An efficacy trial with gay and bisexual men. *AIDS and Behavior, 1,* 137-154.

Scott, J., Conner, D., Venohr, I., Gade, G., McKenzie, M., Kramer, A., et al. (2004). Effectiveness of a group outpatient visit model for chronically ill older HMO members: A 2-year randomized trial of the Cooperative Health Care Clinic. *Journal of the American Geriatric Society, 52,* 1463-1470.

Semansky, R., Koyanagi, C., & Vandivort-Warren, R. (2003). Behavior health screening policies in Medicaid programs nationwide. *Psychiatric Services, 54*(5), 736-739.

Simonian, S. & Tarnowski. (2001). Utility of the Pediatric Symptom Checklist for behavioral screening of disadvantaged children. *Child Psychiatry and Human Development, 31*(4), 269-278.

Steinman, K., Steinman, M., & Steinman, T. (2003). Disease management programs in the geriatric setting: Practical considerations. *Disease Management and Health Outcomes, 11*(6), 363-374.

Tinkelman, D. & Schwartz, A. (2004). School-based asthma disease management. *Journal of Asthma, 41*(4), 455-462.

Tolson, E., Reid, W., & Garvin, C. (2002). *Generalist practice: A task-centered approach.* New York: Columbia University Press.

U.S. Department of Health and Human Services, Substance Abuse and Mental Health Administration, National Clearinghouse for Alcohol and Drug Information (2004). *Substance abuse among older adults: Treatment Improvement Protocol (TIP) Series 26: Appendix B—Tools.* Retrieved May 9, 2005, from www .health.org/govpubs/bkd250/26k.aspx.

U.S. Preventive Services Task Force (2004). *Screening and behavioral counseling interventions in primary care to reduce alcohol misuse.* Retrieved May 23, 2005, from www.preventiveservices.ahrq.gov.

Wallace, K. (1997). Analysis of recent literature concerning relaxation and imagery interventions with cancer pain. *Cancer Nursing, 20*(2), 79-87.

Weaver, H. (2005). *Explorations in cultural competence: Journeys to the four directions.* Belmont, CA: Thomson/Brooks/Cole.

WALMYR Publishing Company (2005). *Sample scales.* Retrieved May 2, 2005, from www.walmyr.com/samples.html.

Chapter 6

Arches, J. (2001). Powerful partnerships. *Journal of Community Practice, 9*(2), 15-30.

Auslander, W., Haire-Joshu, D., Houston, C., Williams, J., & Krebill, H. (2000). The short-term impact of a health promotion program for low-income African American women. *Research on Social Work Practice, 10*(1), 78-97.

Bowie, S. & Rocha, C. (2004). The promise of public housing as a community-based model of health care. *Health & Social Work, 29*(4), 335-340.

Cameron, J. & Mauksch, L. (2002). Collaborative family health care in an uninsured primary care population: Stages of integration. *Family, Systems and Health, 20,* 343-363.

Chillag, K., Bartholow, K., Cordeiro, J., Swanson, S., Patterson, J., Stebbins, S., et al. (2002). Factors affecting the delivery of HIV/AIDS prevention programs by community-based organizations. *AIDS Education and Prevention, 14*(3/ Supp.), 27-37.

Dunlop, J. M. & Angell, G. (2001). Inside-outside: boundary-spanning challenges in building rural health coalitions. *Professional Development, 4*(1), 40-48.

Dziegielewski, S. & Jacinto, G. (2004). New horizons: Health and wellness. In S. Dziegielewski, *The changing face of health care social work: Professional practice in an era of managed care* (2nd ed., pp. 294-315). New York: Springer Publishing.

Franklin, C. & Corcoran, J. (2000). Preventing adolescent pregnancy: A review of programs and practices. *Social Work, 45,* 40-52.

Galambos, C. (2003). Building healthy environments: Community- and consumer-based initiatives. *Health & Social Work, 28*(3), 171-174.

Gellis, Z. (2001). Social work perceptions of transformational and transactional leadership in health care. *Social Work Research, 25*(10), 17-25.

Gibelman, M. (2003). *Navigating human service organizations.* Chicago, IL: Lyceum Books.

Glisson, C. (2000). Organizational climate and culture. In R. Patti (Ed.), *Handbook of social welfare management* (pp. 195-218). Thousand Oaks, CA: Sage.

Hardina, D. (2002). *Analyzing skills for community organization practice.* New York: Columbia University Press.

Hatchett, B. & Duran, D. (2002). An approach to community outreach in the 21st century. *Journal of Community Practice, 10*(2), 37-51.

King, N. & Ross, A. (2003). Professional identities and interprofessional relationships: Evaluation of collaborative community schema. *Social Work in Health Care, 38*(2), 51-72.

Kreuter, M., Lezin, N., & Young, L. (2000). Evaluating community-based collaboration mechanisms: Implication for practitioners. *Health Promotion Practice, 1*(1), 49-63.

Kreuter, M., Lukwago, S., Bucholtz, D., Clark, E., & Sanders-Thompson, V. (2002). Achieving cultural appropriateness in health promotion programs: Targeted and tailored approaches. *Health Education & Behavior, 30*(2), 133-146.

Lowenberg, F., Dolgoff, R., & Harrington, D. (2000). *Ethical decisions for social work practice* (6th ed.). Itasca, IL: Peacock Publishers, Inc.

Mason, J., Edlow, M., Lear, M., Scoppetta, S., Walther, V., Epstein, I., et al. (2001). Screening for psychosocial risk in an urban prenatal clinic: A retrospective practice-based research study. *Social Work in Health Care, 33*(3/4), 33-52.

Monahan, D. (2001). Teen pregnancy prevention outcomes: Implications for social work practice. *Families in Society: The Journal of Contemporary Human Services, 82*(2), 127-135.

National Resource Center for Family Centered Practice (2004). *Patch approach.* Retrieved September 9, 2004, from www.uiowa.edu/-nrchfp/publications/patch_approach.shtml.

Netting, F., Kettner, P., & McMurty, S. (2004). *Social work macro practice* (3rd ed.). Boston, MA: Allyn and Bacon, Pearson Education Inc.

Paz, J. (2000). Latinos and HIV. In L.Vincent (Ed.), *HIV/AIDS at Year 2000* (pp. 97-106). Boston, MA: Allyn & Bacon.

Poole, D. & Van Hook, M. (1997). Retooling for community health partnerships in primary care. *Health & Social Work, 22*(1), 2-5.

Powell, J., Dosser, D., Handron, D., McCammon, S., Temkin, M., & Kaufman, M. (1999). Challenges of interdisciplinary collaboration: A faculty consortium's initial attempts to model collaborative practice. *Journal of Community Practice, 6*(2), 27-48.

Ramos, R. & Ferreira-Pinto, J. (2002). A model for capacity-building in AIDS prevention programs. *AIDS Education and Prevention, 14*(3), 196-206.

Rank, M. & Hutchison, W. (2000). An analysis of leadership within the social work profession. *Journal of Social Work Education, 36*(3), 487-502.

Roby, J. & Woodson, K. (2004). An evaluation of a breast-feeding education intervention among Spanish-speaking families. *Social Work in Health Care, 40*(1), 15-31.

Rosenberg, G. & Holden, G. (1997). The role of social work in improving quality of life in the community. *Social Work in Health Care, 25*(1/2), 9-22.

Shortell, S., Zukoski, A., Alexander, J., Bazzoli, G., Conrad, D., Kasnain-Wynia, R., et al. (2002). Evaluating partnerships for community health improvement: Tracking the footprints. *Journal of Health Politics, Policy and Law, 27*(1), 49-77.

Thompson, M., Minkler, M., Bell, J., Rose, K., & Butler, L. (2003). Facilitators of well-functioning consortia: National Healthy Start Program lessons. *Health & Social Work, 28*(3), 185-196.

Weaver, H. (2005). *Explorations in cultural competence: Journeys to the four directions.* Belmont, CA: Thomson/Brooks/Cole.

Chapter 7

Alter, C. & Murty, S. (1997). Logic modeling: A tool for teaching practice evaluation. *Journal of Social Work Education, 33*(1), 103-118.

Auslander, G. (2000). Outcomes of social work interventions in health care settings. *Social Work in Health Care, 31*(2), 31-46.

Berkman, B. & Maramaldi, P. (2001). Use of standardized measures in agency based reseach and practice. *Social Work in Health Care, 34*(1/2), 115-129.

Bloom, M., Fischer, J., & Orme, J. (2003). *Evaluating practice: Guidelines for the accountable professional* (4th ed.). Boston, MA: Allyn & Bacon.

Chernesky, R. & Grube, B. (2000). Examining the HIV/AIDS case management process. *Health & Social Work, 25*(4), 243-253.

Corcoran, K. & Fischer, J. (2001). *Measures for clinical practice: A sourcebook* (3rd ed.). New York: The Free Press.

Corcoran, K., Gingerich, W., & Briggs, H. (2003). Practice evaluation: Setting goals and monitoring change. In H. Briggs & K. Corcoran (Eds.), *Social work practice: Treating common client problems* (pp. 66-84). Chicago: Lyceum Press.

Netting, F., Kettner, P., & McMurty, S. (2004). *Social work macro practice* (3rd ed.). Boston, MA: Allyn & Bacon, Pearson Education Inc.

Nugent, B. 2000. Single case design visual analysis procedures for use in practice evaluation. *Journal of Social Service Research, 37*(4), 39-75.

Patterson, D. & Basham, R. (2005). Single system designs. In D. Patterson & Basham, R. (Eds.), *Data analysis with spreadsheets* (pp. 123-145). Boston, MA: Pearson/Allyn Bacon.

Patton, M. (2002). *Qualitative research & evaluation methods* (3rd ed.). Thousand Oaks, CA: Sage.

Rock, B. & Cooper, M. (2000). Social work in primary care: A demonstration student unit utilizing practice research. *Social Work in Health Care, 31*(1), 1-15.

Rossi, P., Freeman, H., & Lipsey, M. (1999). *Evaluation: A systematic approach* (6th ed.) Thousand Oaks, CA: Sage.

Weaver, H. (2005). *Explorations in cultural competence: Journeys to the four directions.* Belmont, CA: Thomson/Brooks/Cole.

Zlotnick, J. & Galambos, C. (2004). Evidence-based practices in health care: Social work responsibilities. *Health & Social Work, 29*(4), 259-261.

Appendix A

Centers for Disease Control (2001). *HIV/AIDS Surveillance Report, 13*(1), 1-41.

Centers for Disease Control, National Center for Health Statistics (2002). *Health: United States.* Retrieved February 23, 2005, from www.cdc.gov/nchs/data/hos/hos04trend.pdf.

Church Health Center (2005). *Connecting minds, bodies and spirits.* Retrieved April 21, 2005, from www.churchhealthcenter.org/html.

Cunningham, M. & Zayas, L (2002). Reducing depression in pregnancy: Designing multimodal interventions. *Social Work, 47*(2), 114-124.

Ginsburg, L. (Ed.). (2005) *Social work in rural communities* (4th ed.). Washington, DC: Council on Social Work Education.

Hope House (2005). *Because no child should be without hope.* Retrieved May 21, 2005, from www.hopehousedaycare.org/HIV-AIDS_fact_sheet.htm.

Letteney, S. & LaPorte, H (2005). Deconstructing stigma: Perceptions of HIV-seropositive mothers and their disclosure to children. *Social Work in Health Care, 38*(3), 105-123.

Owens, S (2003). African American women living with HIV/AIDS: Families as sources of support and of stress. *Social Work, 48*(2), 163-170.

Pistella, C., Bonati, F., & Mihalic, S. (2000). Rural women's perceptions of community prenatal care systems: An empowerment strategy. *Social Work in Health Care, 11*(4), 75-87.

Roby, J. & Woodson, K. (2004). An evaluation of breast-feeding education intervention among Spanish-speaking families. *Social Work in Health Care, 40*(1), 15-31.

U.S. Census Bureau (2001). *Current Population Reports 2000: The Latino population in the United States.* Washington, DC: U.S. Department of Commerce.

Van Loon, R., Borkin, R., & Steffen, J. (2002). Health care experiences and preferences of uninsured workers. *Health & Social Work, 27*(1), 17-26.

Winston, C. (2003). African American grandmothers parenting grandchildren orphaned by AIDS: Grieving and coping with loss. *Illness, Crisis & Loss, 11*(4), 350-362.

Index

Page numbers followed by the letter "f" indicate figures; those followed by the letter "t" indicate tables.

HIV/AIDS *(continued)*
exemplar, 202-203
as focus area for health care, 26
Latino prevention program,
159-160
process evaluation, 188-189
race and, 33t
responding to children's needs,
202-203
telephone conferences, 100
Web sites, 212-213, 215
HMOs. *See* Health maintenance
organizations (HMOs)
Hogg, 72
Holden, G., 86, 89
Homework, 122
Hope House, 202-203
Hospitals
American Association of Hospital
Social Workers, 88
early patient discharge, 5, 10
excess of empty beds, 4
medical social workers, 88-89
Host setting
defined, 90, 103, 179
organizational relationships, 151,
152
Houston, C., 99, 170-171
Hudson Clinical Anxiety Scale, 186
Hudson Short-Form Assessment
Scales, 118, 220
Hull House, 89
Human Genome Project, 100,
218-219
Hyodo, 79
Hypertension
as chronic illness, 39, 40
defined, 47
management of, 45
screening programs, 98

Illness. *See* Disease
Immigrants
acculturation, 72-75
diversity of health care consumers,
27-28
Medicaid exclusions, 42
Improvement and Protection Act of
2000, 99

Incidence
defined, 47
of HIV/AIDS, 37-38
Individualized rating scales
defined, 196
in single-system design, 184
Infant mortality
defined, 104
rates of, 28-29
social work in health care, 87
Institute of Medicine, 91
Insurance. *See* Health insurance
Interactive leadership, 172
Interdisciplinary
care coordination, 144
collaboration. *See* Interdisciplinary
collaboration
defined, 84, 104
in disease management, 125
health care teams, 139-142
multidisciplinary vs., 84
organizational relationships, 152
primary care collaboration, 94
professional differences for
intervention, 141
Interdisciplinary collaboration
defined, 179
by teams, 139, 152-154
Internet for health care information,
99-100, 132
Interventions
CBT. *See* Cognitive-behavioral
intervention
complementary and alternative,
130-131
crisis intervention, 128-130
evidence-based. See Evidence-based
interventions
professional differences, 141
small groups, 132-137
Interviewing for understanding
community, 158-160, 161

Jacinto, G., 169-170
Jansson, B., 138
Johns Hopkins Medical School, 87
Johnson, Robert Woods, 205
Judeo-Christian
sexual orientation, 71
traditions, 58

Public organizations
corporation monopoly, 11
defined, 24
organizational structure, 150

Qualitative data analysis, 194
Quantitative data analysis, 194

Race
asthma and, 33t
chronic illnesses by racial
categories, 33, 33t
diabetes and, 33t, 35-36
of health care consumers, 29
HIV and, 33t
uninsured/underinsured, 43-44
Referrals, 84
Reflection, communication technique,
114
Reframing, 122
Reisen, C., 74
Religion. *See* Spiritual orientation
Renal
defined, 47
diabetes impact, 34
Rhee, C.-W., 99
Risk factor
defined, 47
of hypertension, 39, 40
of obesity, 39-40
Roby, J., 201-202
Rocha, C., 164
Rock, B., 17, 182
Roffman, R., 100
Role-playing, 122
Rosenberg, G., 86, 89
Ross, A., 153-154

Santeria
beliefs of, 64
defined, 81
SARS (self-anchored rating scale), 185
Schema
cognitive-behavioral theory, 112,
126, 127
defined, 112, 146

Schilder, A., 72
Screening programs
assessment tools and instruments,
117-119
as secondary prevention, 98
Secondary prevention
defined, 104, 169, 179
purpose of, 98
Self-anchored rating scale (SARS),
185
Self-determination, 138, 173
Self-monitoring, 127-128
Self-talk, 112, 127
Sequela
defined, 47
of diabetes, 34, 35
diabetes impact, 33-34
Settings for health care
different structures, 86
host setting. *See* Host setting
Sexual orientation
cultural background, 55, 70-72
defined, 71
terms, 71-72
SF-36 assessment tool, 117-118,
219-220
Shadid, Michael, 7
Sickle cell anemia group intervention,
135-136
Sikkema, L., 100
Simonian, S., 119
Single-system design
applicability, 182
before-and-after designs, 183,
184-185
data analysis, 186-188, 187f
data collection, 184-186
defined, 197
designing, 183
goal attainment scales. *See* Goal
attainment scales (GAS)
target issues, 184
in university-care collaboration,
182-183
visualization, 186-188, 187f
Small groups for intervention, 132-137
Social rules and values
assessment topics and questions,
222
cultural background, 55
cultural competence, 75-79